More with Less

INTERNATIONAL HUMANITARIAN AFFAIRS

Kevin M. Cahill, M.D., series editor

More with Less

Disasters in an Era of Diminishing Resources

EDITED BY **KEVIN M. CAHILL, M.D.**

A JOINT PUBLICATION **OF FORDHAM UNIVERSITY PRESS** AND
THE CENTER FOR INTERNATIONAL HUMANITARIAN COOPERATION
NEW YORK 2012

Fordham University Press has no responsibility for
the persistence or accuracy of URLs for external or
third-party Internet websites referred to in this
publication and does not guarantee that any content
on such websites is, or will remain, accurate or
appropriate.

Fordham University Press also publishes its books in a
variety of electronic formats. All of the books in the
International Humanitarian Book Series are available
in electronic format. Some content that appears in
print may not be available in electronic books.

Library of Congress Cataloging-in-Publication Data

More with less : disasters in an era of diminishing
resources / edited by Kevin M. Cahill.
        p. cm. — (International humanitarian affairs)
    "A joint publication of Fordham University Press
and the Center for International Humanitarian
Cooperation."
    Includes bibliographical references and index.
    ISBN 978-0-8232-5017-2 (cloth : alk. paper)—
ISBN 978-0-8232-5018-9 (pbk. : alk. paper)
    1. Humanitarian assistance. 2. Disaster relief.
3. International relief. I. Cahill, Kevin M. II. Center
for International Humanitarian Cooperation.
    HV553.M668 2012
    363.34'8—dc23
                                        2012020966

Printed in the United States of America.

14 13 12   5 4 3 2 1

First edition

*All royalties from this book go to the training of humanitarian
workers.*

For Peter Hansen
Scholar, Diplomat, Colleague, and Friend

CONTENTS

Preparedness

Response

Entrepreneurial Approaches

Disaster risk is increasing globally. Over the past decade, disasters caused by natural hazards have affected more than 2.2 billion people and killed over 840,000. The economic cost of these disasters was at least $891 billion. These are losses to countries' welfare and to individual livelihoods and future.

In 2011 we witnessed a sequence of consecutive disasters caused by earthquakes, tsunamis and weather-related events. At the same time, the world has gone through a financial crisis that has plunged many countries into recession and negatively affected the economic growth of others. This crisis has led to intense scrutiny of expenditure and priorities. Calls for more efficiency and "burden sharing" in international and national cooperation are frequently heard.

During my Presidency of the Sixty-Sixth Session of the United Nations General Assembly, I have traveled to disaster sites and seen the effects of the tsunami in Japan, the devastation of famine in Somalia, and the largest refugee camp in the world in Kenya.

Donors who finance humanitarian relief recognize the risks and the lack of sustainability of their increasing expenditure for humanitarian situations. This pressure on resources and on vulnerability motivates us to find new solutions, rethink our strategies, and redefine our actions to ensure that every dollar spent in aid—whether development and humanitarian—will result in more resilient and sustainable cities, communities, and nations.

The positive news is that preventive action is less expensive than cure. Reducing disaster risk is about ensuring that our investments in development are not washed away when the next flood or tsunami occurs. Sometimes it's about making the right decision at the right time—decisions such as not building a school, hospital, or bridge in harm's way. Reducing disaster risk is also about being innovative, working in partnership, and striking new alliances with all relevant actors, including the private sector and civil society.

In light of their disproportionate losses, better understanding is needed about the lives of girls and women before, during, and after disaster. A gendered perspective on preparedness, relief, recovery and mitigation is essential for effective action and will provide insight into how globalization, urbanization, and environmental degradation affect women's disaster vulnerability in rich as well as poor nations. Gender relations clearly play a role in the political economy of disaster; in organizational relief and response; in community leadership and mobilization; in household preparation and family recovery; and in survival strategies in disaster-resilient communities. Specific guidelines are essential for integrating gender issues into the preparedness activities for disaster planning, as well as for ensuring provision of gender-fair assistance.

I applaud the courage of those countries that have already taken steps toward reducing disaster risk and thus saving lives and ensuring that money is spent wisely. Experience has shown that investing in disaster-risk reduction can result in significant economic returns. A number of countries have also invested in preventive measures which have yielded multiple benefits, not least in saving many lives and livelihoods.

Reducing disaster risk should not be seen as an additional expenditure, but rather an investment for a safer and more resilient world. It also empowers people to face the challenges of disaster more effectively. We must strengthen our commitment toward more preventive approaches in order to ensure that our development investments are secured—not destroyed in a matter of seconds when the next calamity happens. Countries may best meet this challenge by considering a global action plan to reduce disaster risk. This will be a reassuring leap forward to meet the challenges of the coming decades.

H.E. Nassir Abdulaziz Al-Nasser
President of the Sixty-Sixth Session
of the United Nations General Assembly

ACKNOWLEDGMENTS

This is the twelfth volume in the International Humanitarian Affairs Book Series, seven of which have been published by Fordham University Press. A number of the books have gone into multiple reprintings, and new editions; seven have been translated into French. All of the texts—whether written solely by me, or based on chapters contributed by experts from around the world—have been intended to strengthen the emerging discipline of humanitarian action. All royalties from the series have been applied to the training of a future generation of humanitarian workers.

With deep gratitude I acknowledge the generosity of the contributors to this volume. From incredibly busy schedules they somehow carved out time to create chapters that would help focus global attention on a critical problem: how to prepare for, and respond to, disasters in an era when many traditional donors are facing their own economic crises.

My main assistant in the editing process was Jenna Felz of the Institute of International Humanitarian Affairs (IIHA) at Fordham University. Alycia Kravitz and Denis Cahill helped edit several chapters. Mr. Peter Hansen generously shared his vast knowledge of the United Nations and humanitarian community to the benefit of both the Introduction and other chapters in this text. Mr. Fredric Nachbaur and the staff of Fordham University Press provided a level of publishing expertise that I have come to admire as the series has developed.

The Fordham University family supported this project from its inception. I am particularly grateful to President Joseph McShane, S.J., to Provost Stephen Freedman, and to the Executive Director of the IIHA, Brendan Cahill.

Finally, the Foreword to this volume was contributed by H.E. Nassir Abdulaziz Al-Nasser, the President of the United Nations General Assembly, Sixty-Sixth Session. I have had the privilege of serving as his Chief Advisor on Humanitarian and Public Health Issues. He identified "Disaster Preparedness and Response" as one of the four main objectives of his tenure, and this book is intended to honor that commitment and be a permanent part of the legacy of his Presidency.

From the halls of the United Nations to a sprawling refugee camp in Kenya, from the bombed-out remains of Mogadishu, Somalia, to countless shared meals in New York and Doha, I was fortunate to see the passionate, profound dedication of this most distinguished diplomat. I also was privileged to observe his steady compassion for those in need, his innate decency and modesty, his concern for his staff and, maybe most moving, his joyous love for Aziz and Muna.

BRICs	Brazil, Russia, India, and China
BWIs	Bretton Woods Institutions
CAP	Consolidated Appeals Process (OCHA)
CDC	Centers for Disease Control and Prevention
CERF	Central Emergency Response Fund
CFA	Comprehensive Framework for Action
CGD	Commission on Growth and Development
CSW	commercial sex worker
DAC	Development Assistance Committee
DEC	Disaster Emergency Committee (UK)
DFID	Department for International Development
DRC	Danish Refugee Council
DVI	Disaster Victim Identification
EG	Educate Girls (Rajastani NGO)
G8	Group of Eight
GDACS	Global Disaster Alert and Coordination System
GDP	gross domestic profit
GHD	Good Humanitarian Donorship initiative
GIS	geographic information system
GNI	gross national income
HLTF	High-Level Task Force
ICRC	International Committee of the Red Cross

IDHA   International Diploma in Humanitarian Assistance (Fordham University)

IFRC   International Federation of Red Cross and Red Crescent Societies

IHA   International Humanitarian Affairs (Fordham University)

IIHA   Institute of International Humanitarian Affairs (Fordham University)

IMF   International Monetary Fund

IOC   Intergovernmental Oceanographic Commission

MDG   Millennium Development Goal

MIHA   Masters in International Humanitarian Action (Fordham University)

MSF   Médecins Sans Frontières

NATO   North Atlantic Treaty Organization

NCD   noncommunicable disease

NGO   nongovernmental organization

OCHA   Office for the Coordination of Humanitarian Affairs

ODA   official development assistance

OECD   Organisation for Economic Co-operation and Development

OHCHR   Office of the United Nations High Commissioner for Human Rights

OIC   Organisation of Islamic Cooperation

OSOCC   On-Site Operations Coordination Centre

PGA   President of the United Nations General Assembly

PIH   Partners in Health

R2P   Responsibility to Protect

SBTF   Standby Task Force

SIDS   Small Island Developing States

TEC   Tsunami Evaluation Coalition

UN   United Nations

UNDHA   United Nations Department of Humanitarian Affairs

UNDRO   United Nations Department for Relief Operations

UNESCO   United Nations Educational, Scientific and Cultural Organization

UNGA	United Nations General Assembly
UNHCR	United Nations High Commissioner for Refugees
UNHRC	United Nations Human Rights Council
UNICEF	United Nations Children's Fund
UNISDR	United Nations International Strategy for Disaster Reduction
UNRRA	United Nations Relief and Rehabilitation Agency
UNRWA	United Nations Relief and Works Agency
UNWTO	United Nations World Tourism Organization
USAID	United States Agency for International Development
WEF	World Economic Forum
WFP	World Food Programme
WHO	World Health Organization

INTRODUCTION

KEVIN M. CAHILL, M.D.

Humanitarian workers, if they are to be effective, must be realists. They deal every day with the cruel facts of human suffering, and no amount of rhetoric can alleviate pain or provide sustenance in times of widespread natural or man-made crises. This book reflects the reality that resources available for disaster preparedness and disaster response have been seriously diminished by the current global economic recession.[1] It documents the evolution of global philanthropy, while also examining alternative methods to reduce costs through better preventive programs and suggesting potential sources for additional future funding for relief operations. It is not unrealistic for international humanitarian workers to believe that we can do *More with Less.*

Humanitarian assistance is a discipline that attracts men and women who, in often terrible situations, continue to strive for a better world. They have dreams and visions, values and traditions, that have not been suppressed by many earlier challenges. In fact, improvements in disaster prevention and response have often come *because* of adversity. These improvements—the establishment of accepted standards for health, shelter, food, protection, human rights, education, a code of ethics for workers, and an emerging body of human rights and humanitarian law—have all been realized by learning lessons from past humanitarian missions. They have also, very significantly, been accomplished without abandoning the noble principles of independence, neutrality, and impartiality that are the foundation for our work.

One of the main dangers ahead, it seems to me, is that this very foundation may be destroyed in the name of bureaucratic efficiency and fiscal concerns. If the special role of international humanitarian work is not recognized then it will quickly be subordinated to military and political forces, especially in complex humanitarian crises and conflict situations. It is that concern that motivated me to ask leaders in different disciplines to reflect on how we can do More with Less, and do it in a way that preserves the integrity of international humanitarian assistance.

This book is intended to be a lasting part of the legacy of the President of the United Nations General Assembly (PGA), Sixty-Sixth Session. The PGA, H.E. Nassir Abdulaziz al Nasser, is the senior person in the world's ultimate diplomatic organization. It is in his honor, therefore, that I begin this text by considering the essential role of the United Nations (UN) in managing disasters.

When the UN Charter was drafted in 1945, there was but a single mention of humanitarian affairs. Maybe understandably, in the terrible afterglow of World War II, the Charter focused on human rights and the prevention of conflict. The Charter has, as its foundation, the sovereignty of Member States. International humanitarian action often necessitates cross-border activities in order to offer relief for victims. For that reason, humanitarians also contend that their work warrants respect for a neutral—as opposed to political—space in which they can provide impartial assistance to all in need.

There seems to be an inherent conflict in these views on sovereignty (at least as understood at the birth of the UN) and on intervention (as based on evolving concepts of the obligations of a State toward its citizens). I shall return to this later. Suffice it to note here that the full history of the UN is, fortunately, far more nuanced than the words of the Charter.

While the Charter is almost silent on humanitarian assistance, the deeds of the organization speak for themselves. UN-led relief operations actually predate the final signing of the Charter. The United Nations Relief and Rehabilitation Agency (UNRRA) was its first major international operation, offering critical help across the destroyed landscape of Europe, addressing hunger and other needs of refugees as

World War II was winding down. When the United Nations Children's Fund (UNICEF) was founded in 1946, the "E" stood for Emergency, signifying its orientation to assist children anywhere, even across conflicted borders.

Later, in 1949, the United Nations Relief and Works Agency (UNRWA) was created to serve some 780,000 Palestine refugees who had been displaced in camps across a half-dozen countries. The United Nations High Commissioner for Refugees (UNHCR) was established in 1950 to deal with refugees fleeing as the Iron Curtain descended over Eastern Europe.

As the Cold War ended, and international attention could be focused on the former proxy states of the Big Powers, the UN gradually assumed an even greater role in humanitarian work. UNHCR became a major provider in the Balkan conflicts of the early 1990s. A UN role as coordinator of relief efforts had been formalized by the establishment of a separate United Nations Department for Relief Operations (UNDRO) in 1972. But that mandate was only limited to natural disasters. It was after the Cold War that the United Nations Department of Humanitarian Affairs (DHA) was established in 1991 to address all disasters, all around the world, and regardless of their cause. DHA was succeeded by the Office for the Coordination of Humanitarian Affairs (OCHA) in 1995.

These developments reflected the ability of the international community to be able to better respond to complex humanitarian crises in zones formally under the absolute control of Big Powers. This period of a gradual evolution in our understanding of the nature of sovereignty, and of the tensions that exist between those who favor intervention over the absolute rights of states, is ongoing. The Responsibility to Protect (R2P) thesis has been used to justify various humanitarian interventions, but not without a growing concern about the limits and justification for such actions.

A further development at the UN—that the organization should deliver assistance "as one"—has inevitably increased the involvement of political and military actors in what had previously been solely the humanitarian domain based on principles of independence, neutrality, and impartiality. There are obvious dangers in "coordinating" responses by placing all efforts under one command. Military and political solutions to resolving complex humanitarian crises are the complete inverse of the traditional humanitarian approach. By definition, military and political positions are not neutral or impartial or independent.

The larger, more powerful actors are likely to dominate a response and implement "national interests," particularly those of the major powers. When U.S. Secretary of State Colin Powell said he viewed humanitarian organizations as "force multipliers" for American policies in Iraq, there was widespread alarm in, and rejection by, international humanitarian nongovernmental organizations (NGOs). Nevertheless, pressures for such an approach, resulting in the destruction of humanitarian work as we have known it, are increasing.

The goal of complete coordination of UN activity in complex humanitarian crises may well destroy the very freedom that has made international humanitarian assistance so unique and effective for centuries. There is almost certain to be significant resistance to this approach in the international humanitarian community.

These challenges are complicated by the eroding financial base of traditional support for international disaster relief appeals. The current global economic crisis has put significant strain on many Western nations that have provided the majority of funds for past crises. The Organisation for Economic Co-operation and Development (OECD), the premiere international forum for analyzing development and aid data, has documented significant reductions in official development assistance (ODA) from major donors. There is every expectation on projections for 2012–15 that the downward trend will continue. Some of the reductions in donations for overseas aid from financially affected countries were very striking; for example, Greece and Spain were both down over 35 percent in a single year. The total net ODA fell by 4.5 percent in real terms between 2010 and 2011. It is too early to be certain how the world will respond to future disasters, but the trends are worrying, and there are risks—at least in political rhetoric—of a return to isolationism.

In addition, there are also demographic changes in many Western nations—a growing percentage of the population being elderly or pensioners, and a declining percentage being productive members of the workforce—that are likely to make their governments refocus resources from foreign assistance to domestic needs. Radical change has, however, often presented unexpected opportunities, and there are lights in this dark tunnel.

To date, many of the emerging economic powers—China, Russia, India, the nations of Latin America, and the Middle East—have not been in the financial forefront of disaster relief operations. Perhaps they may have felt isolated—and unwanted—dealing with Western approaches that have so dominated the international appeals process. As the humanitarian community moves forward, it is obvious that it must develop a broader inclusive framework that welcomes all cultures, and respects the values, principles, religions, customs, interests, and legitimate concerns of these new potential donors.

Fundamentally, most people believe there is a universal value system that allows us all—especially in a world of instant communication—to know when other human beings, our brothers and sisters in a global family, are suffering and dying due to natural or man-made disasters. Such a universal value system must be promoted so that all nations feel a responsibility to participate in every humanitarian crisis.

As the donor base changes, there must also be an increased sensitivity to the very real concerns of those who have the impression that international humanitarian intervention mandates can be merely a cover for other political goals. For example, the U.S.–NATO intervention in Libya in 2011 was initially justified on a humanitarian basis, but it quickly evolved into an operation overtly aimed at regime change. It is imperative to keep these actions separate and distinct, or the international community risks fatally tarnishing the ideals of humanitarianism, and also alienating the new donors who must share the burdens of relief as equal and appreciated partners.

There will undoubtedly be other challenges to the present system of funding and directing international humanitarian assistance. Recognizing trends, and trying to deal constructively with the cultures of new donors, will make the transition more palatable. Some of the emerging powers clearly prefer bilateral arrangements for their donations, and this might be construed as weakening the role of the UN. But the reality is that for the past few decades the UN has had a relatively declining role in relief operations, while assuming a more central role for coordination.

In the field, international and local NGOs, and bilateral government aid, are already the dominant forces, and, as suggested above, UN coordination will demand a much more nuanced approach than the current mantra of delivering aid "as one." There are also concerns that some new donors might tie their donations to commercial operations. But is that so different from the current practices of major donors clearly linking their own national interests and geopolitics with relief contributions?

While the world—especially through the UN, hopefully using mediation rather than armed force—may help to avert the terrible disasters of war and conflict, the pace of natural and man-made disasters will surely grow in the foreseeable future. Climate change, deforestation and consequent floods, desertification, earthquakes, tsunamis, typhoons, and hurricanes are a regular part of many human lives. Careful preparation for such disasters will lessen the damage and loss of life. Learning lessons from past crises, applying new technologies, and developing better-trained responders will help when disasters strike.

The realist—and the optimist—in the emerging discipline of humanitarian relief work must be flexible enough to move beyond the traditional boundaries of the profession. As one example of seeking solutions "outside the box," I conclude this book with a section on the potential contributions that entrepreneurs can make to both disaster preparedness and response.

Entrepreneurs approach humanitarian problems using business models—and acumen—and have helped refocus humanitarian visions, dreams, and aspirations. The private sector, using creative organizational skills combined with a willingness to take risks and build productive teams, provides effective operations that large bureaucracies might well emulate. Entrepreneurs can be critical partners in an endeavor that cannot afford to isolate contributors.

At the local level there is also clear evidence that the toll of natural disasters can be reduced by the active participation of civil society. Since they know the strengths and weaknesses of their local communities best they can, for example, help in the demand for safe architectural standards for schools and hospitals. Local groups can establish regional partnerships so that refuge and assistance is more rapidly available in times of crisis.

Disaster preparedness and response is a challenge that can unite mankind—from the UN to national and local governments, from concerned NGOs to every sector of civil society, from businesses to the arts—using volunteers as well as trained professionals to prevent and alleviate so much needless suffering and death. We must—and can—do *More with Less*.

This section offers an overview of the global economy and its impact on international humanitarian assistance. Budgetary cuts are probably inevitable—and certainly understandable—in government programs not directly helpful to a rising number of domestic unemployed dependent on the state for food, health and shelter. Case studies on how a large relief agency, and a proud nation, cope in an era of declining resources follow. Both offer hope for eventual recovery, but history indicates that the levels of charitable giving following any prolonged recession are slow to return to earlier levels. Nevertheless, as the final chapter indicates, the resilience of the downtrodden, and promoting local capacity, offers a positive path ahead.

Globalization, Growth, Poverty, Governance, and Humanitarian Assistance

DOMINICK SALVATORE

This chapter examines humanitarian assistance to populations afflicted by major natural and man-made disasters in the broader context of the evolution of world poverty in our rapidly globalizing world. Although many natural disasters can and do occur in rich and poor countries alike, they have been, and are generally, more common in the latter than the former, and it is in poor countries that they inflict the most suffering—thus creating the greatest need for humanitarian assistance. When a rich country faces a natural disaster (as for example, Japan from the earthquake and tsunami in 2011), it generally has adequate resources to come to the rescue of the afflicted populations. When the disaster occurs in a poor country on the other hand, it usually leads to a greater human tragedy and much greater suffering because the poor country usually does not have the resources or the ability to deal with the crisis, especially if it is man-made, as in the case of civil wars or other forms of internal strife. It is in these cases that humanitarian assistance is most needed and urgent.

In short, poor countries seem more prone to natural, but especially to man-made, disasters, and are much less prepared to deal with them, thus necessitating large-scale outside assistance. Rapid growth and development is crucial to reduce the occurrence of man-made disasters and to make the nation better prepared and able to deal with them, as well as with natural disasters when they occur. Both of these goals can be achieved if a poor country grows and develops rapidly and reduces its level of poverty. This chapter examines humanitarian assistance in this broader context.

I will first examine how globalization has affected growth and development during the most recent period of rapid globalization that started in the early 1980s, and how growth and development in turn has affected and affects the level and extent of poverty in developing countries. Then, I will examine what the United Nations (UN), the World Bank, the International Monetary Fund, and other international aid organizations, as well as rich nations individually, can do to facilitate and encourage more rapid growth and development. I will also focus on how world governance can be changed to allow a poor country to receive a greater share of the benefits emanating from rapid globalization as well as to empower poor people everywhere so as to reduce the occurrence of man-made disasters and to be better able to deal with them and with natural disasters when they do occur.

The Growth Report

In 2008, the high-powered Commission on Growth and Development (CGD) published *The Growth Report*, which provided an in-depth analysis of the common characteristics of the thirteen high-growth economies during the postwar period. The high-growth countries are defined as those that achieved an average real growth rate of at least 7 percent per year over a period of at least twenty-five years from 1950 to 2005.[1]

Although the CGD could not find any unique blueprint for ensuring high growth, it found that the high-growth countries shared five common characteristics. They all:

1. fully "exploited" the world economy;

2. maintained macroeconomic stability;

3. mustered high rates of savings and investment;

4. let markets allocate resources;

5. had committed, credible and capable governments.

While not specifically mentioned by name, globalization and international competitiveness seem to be essential characteristics of a high-growth strategy. Characteristic 1 (fully "exploited" the world economy) means globalization and characteristic 4 (let markets allocate resources) is an essential ingredient of international competitiveness and growth.

Globalization of Production and Labor Markets

There is a strong trend toward globalization in production and in labor markets in the world economy today. For those firms and nations that do take advantage of this trend the results are increased efficiency, competitiveness, and growth. Global corporations play a crucial role in the process of globalization. These are companies that are run by an international team of managers, have research and production facilities in many countries, use parts and components from the cheapest sources around the world, sell their products globally, and are owned by stockholders throughout the world who finance their operations. More and more corporations today operate on the belief that their survival requires them to be one of a handful of global corporations in their sector. This is true in the automobile, steel, telecommunications, and aircraft industries, and for companies that produce computers, consumer electronics, chemicals, drugs, and many other products and services.

One important form of globalization in the area of production is outsourcing, or the foreign "sourcing" of inputs. There is practically no major product today that does not have some foreign inputs. Foreign sourcing is often not a choice made by corporations in the hope of earning higher profits, but simply a requirement for those that wish to remain competitive. Firms that do not look abroad for cheaper inputs risk not being able to compete in world—and even domestic—markets. Such low cost, offshore purchase of inputs is likely to continue to expand rapidly in the future and is being fostered by joint ventures, licensing arrangements, and other nonequity collaborative arrangements.

Foreign sourcing can be regarded as manufacturing's new *international* economies of scale in today's global economy. Just as companies were forced to rationalize operations within each country during the 1980s, they now face the challenge of integrating their operations for their entire system of manufacturing around the world in order to take advantage of the new international economies of scale. The most successful multinational corporations are those that focus on their core competencies that are indispensable to their competitive position over subsequent product generations and "outsource" all the rest from outside suppliers.

Even more dramatic than globalization in production is the globalization of labor markets. Work that was previously done in the United States and other industrial countries is now often done much more cheaply in some emerging markets. This is the case not only for low-skill, assembly-line jobs, but also for jobs requiring advanced computer and engineering skills. In fact, a truly competitive global labor force has been developing that is willing and able to do their jobs most efficiently at the lowest possible cost. Even service industries, such as making airline reservations, processing tickets, and answering calls to toll-free numbers are not immune to global job competition. Highly skilled and professional people are not spared from global competition either.

Workers in advanced countries are raising strong objections to the transfer of skilled jobs abroad. Nevertheless, companies in all advanced countries are outsourcing more and more of their work to emerging markets in order to bring or keep costs down and remain internationally competitive. In the future, more and more work will simply be done in those emerging markets best equipped to do a particular job most economically. If governments in advanced nations tried to restrict the flow of work abroad to protect domestic jobs, their firms would risk losing international competitiveness and they may end up having to move all of their operations abroad.

Globalization in production and labor markets is thus important and inevitable—important because it increases efficiency and inevitable because international competition requires it. Besides the well-known static gains from specialization in production and trade, globalization leads to even more important dynamic gains from extending the scale of operation to the entire world and from the more efficient utilization of capital and technology of domestic resources at home and abroad.

Globalization, Economic Growth, and Development

Growth is the most important economic goal of countries today. The best available measure of growth in standards of living that also allows comparisons across countries is in terms of purchasing power parity (PPP) per capita incomes. This takes into account and makes the proper adjustment for all the reasons (such as an undervalued exchange rate and nonmarket production) that usually lead to the underestimation of the true per capita income of developing nations with respect to that of advanced nations. Since we are interested in examining the effect of globalization on growth and development, we will compare the growth of real PPP per capita incomes in various countries and regions of the world since the early 1980s, which is usually taken as the most recent period of rapid globalization, with the two decades (1960–80) before it. Of course, the rate of growth and development of a nation depends not only on globalization but also on many other domestic factors, such as political stability, improvements in education and labor skills, increasing the rate of investment and absorption of new technologies, reducing the rate of population growth, and so on. But globalization is certainly a crucial ingredient for growth.

For example, no one forced China to open up to the world economy, but without such an opening China would not have received the huge inflows of capital and technology that it needed. It would not have been able to increase its exports to the rest of the world so dramatically and thus would not have been able to achieve its spectacular rates of growth of the past two decades. A possibly strong positive correlation between globalization and growth does not, of course, establish causality, but it would refute the assertion on the part of the antiglobal groups that globalization has hampered growth and caused increased inequalities between advanced and developing countries during the past three decades.

Table 1 below gives the growth of the weighted yearly average real PPP (with base 2005) per capita income in various regions and countries of the world in the 1960–80, 1980–2000, and 2000–10 periods. From the table we see that East Asia and Pacific did well during the 1960–80 period and very well since then. The former communist countries of Europe and Central Asia performed poorly during the second period (no data was available for the first period) as a result of the economic collapse associated with the fall of communism and the required economic restructuring that followed it, but grew very rapidly during the third period. Latin America did reasonably well during the first and third periods, but per capita incomes were practically stagnant during the second period (considered the "lost" decades for growth and development) because of political and economic crises. The Middle East and North Africa did well during the first and third periods, but badly during the second period because of political turmoil and wars. South Asia grew at an average rate half as high as East Asia and the Pacific during the 1980–2000 period and at two-thirds that rate during 2000–10. Sub-Saharan Africa did not do well during the first period and actu-

Table 1. Weighted Yearly Average Real PPP per Capita Income Growth in Various Regions, 1960–80, 1980–2000, and 2000–10

REGION	1960–80	1980–2000	2000–10
East Asia and Pacific	2.9	6.1	8.6
Europe and Central Asia	—	1.1	5.2
Latin America and Caribbean	3.1	0.1	2.6
Middle East and North Africa	3.2	0.2	2.9
South Asia	0.6	3.0	5.9
Sub-Saharan Africa	1.3	−0.6	2.5
Developing world	2.1	3.1	5.1
High-income countries	3.9	2.3	1.1

Source: World Bank, *World Development Indicators*, various issues.

ally became poorer during the second period because of political instability, wars, droughts, and the HIV virus, but managed an average growth of 2.5 percent from 2000 to 2010.

The developing world as a whole did reasonably well during the first period, better during the second period, and best during the third period. Overall, only Asia grew faster than industrialized countries and sharply reduced inequalities vis-à-vis industrialized countries, as a group, during the 1980–2000 period. Europe and Central Asia, the Middle East and North Africa, as well as Latin America, did poorly during the second period, so that inequalities increased with respect to high-income countries, but did better during the third period. Sub-Saharan Africa actually became poorer in an absolute sense during the second period, and so it fell further behind advanced countries and other developing countries during the second period, but it recovered some of the lost ground in the third period.

Table 2 shows more directly the correlation between globalization and growth. It shows that the growth of real per capita (PPP) gross domestic profit (GDP) increased sharply in each decade from 1960 to 2010 for the developing countries that globalized (i.e., those for which the ratio of international trade and international financial flows to GDP increased) and far exceeded the average growth of rich countries and that of the nonglobalizers. The growth of rich countries was very high and much higher than that of both the globalizers and nonglobalizers during the decade of the 1960s, but it declined in each subsequent decade. The growth of nonglobalizers increased from the decade of the 1960s to the decade of the 1970s, but then it declined sharply during

Table 2. Weighted Yearly Average Real PPP per Capita Income Growth in Rich Countries, Globalizers, and Nonglobalizers, in the 1960s, 1970s, 1980s, 1990s, and 2000s

GROUP OF COUNTRIES	1960S	1970S	1980S	1990S	2000S
Rich countries	4.7	3.1	2.3	2.2	1.1
Globalizers	1.4	2.9	3.5	5.0	5.0
Nonglobalizers	2.4	3.3	0.8	1.4	2.3

Sources: Dollar and Kraay (2001) and World Bank, *World Development Indicators*, various issues.

the 1980s; it was very low during the 1990s, but then it increased during the 2000–10 period (and it even exceeded the growth of the rich countries). It seems that growth can be rapid without liberalization and globalization at the beginning of the growth process, but as the nation develops, economic efficiency associated with liberalization and globalization becomes increasingly important.

Although there is no perfect correspondence between nonglobalizers and the poorest countries in the world, most nonglobalizers do include most of the poorest countries in the world. Thus, inequalities in per capita incomes and standards of living did increase between nonglobalizers on the one hand and globalizers and the rich countries on the other during the 1980s and 1990s. But the reason for this increased inequality cannot be attributed to globalization as such. Indeed, it was the globalizers that grew fastest during the 1980s and 1990s, while the nonglobalizers stagnated or regressed. Thus, the only (but still serious) criticism that can be levied against globalization, as a process, is that it did not permit the poorest countries of the world to also participate in the tremendous benefits in terms of economic efficiency and growth in living standards that it made possible. This is a far cry, however, from globalization being itself the cause of the increased inequalities between the rich and the globalizing developing countries on the one hand and the poorest and nonglobalizing developing nations on the other during the past three decades, as claimed by the opponents of globalization. During the 2000s, the nonglobalizers, as a group, grew faster than the rich countries and reduced relative income inequalities vis-à-vis the rich countries (but fell further behind vis-à-vis the globalizers).

Globalization and Poverty

Another important question that needs to be answered is what effect globalization has had on actual world poverty at both the country and individual levels. Depending on how we choose to measure relative poverty, however, we get dramatically different results.

One way to measure the evolution of relative poverty is to measure the change in the number of times that the income per capita in the

United States exceeds the income per capita in the world's poorest country, in the tenth-poorest country, or in the twenty poorest countries, as compared with the twenty richest countries in the world over time. Based on this measure, the United Nations (2011[a]), World Bank (2002), and many left-leaning intellectuals such as Pritchett (1997) and Stiglitz (2002) have asserted that globalization caused or resulted in increased income inequalities and poverty in the poorest developing countries over the past decades.

The data presented in Table 3 can shed light on this. The second column of the table shows that the ratio of real PPP per capita income in the United States relative to the poorest country (Lesotho) was 48.3 in 1960, 47.1 (Lesotho) in 1970, 47.4 (Tanzania) in 1980, 51.6 (Tanzania) in 1990, 73.3 (Sierra Leone) in 2000, and 151.7 (Democratic Republic of the Congo) in 2010. Thus, according to this measure, world income inequalities have indeed increased significantly from 1970 to 2010. To avoid the problem of outliers, however, the third column of Table 3 shows that the ratio of real per capita PPP income in the United States relative to the tenth-poorest country (Guinea) was 27.6 in 1960, 31.0 (Nigeria) in 1970, 31.3 (Bhutan) in 1980, 32.5 (Burundi) in 1990, 44.6 (Zambia) in 2000, and 51.1 (Guinea) in 2010. Thus, again, inequalities seem to have increased from 1960 to 2010. Finally, the same general conclusion can be reached from the last column of Table 3 (except for a

Table 3. Ratio of Real PPP per Capita Income in Rich and Poor Countries, 1960–2010

YEAR	IN U.S. RELATIVE TO POOREST COUNTRY	IN U.S. RELATIVE TO 10TH POOREST COUNTRY	IN THE 20 RICHEST COUNTRIES RELATIVE TO THE 20 POOREST COUNTRIES
1960	48.3	27.6	23.0
1970	47.1	31.0	26.2
1980	47.4	31.3	25.7
1990	51.6	32.5	30.8
2000	73.3	44.6	36.3
2010	151.7	51.1	43.3

Sources: Bhalla (2002) and World Bank, *World Development Indicators*, various issues.

Table 4. World Poverty: Number and Percentage of People Living on Less than $1.25 per Day, 1981–2008

REGION/NUMBER OF POOR PEOPLE	1981	1993	2008
East Asia and Pacific	1,096.5	870.8	284.4
China	835.1	632.7	173.0
Eastern Europe and Central Asia	8.2	13.7	2.2
Latin America and Caribbean	43.3	52.5	36.8
Middle East and North Africa	16.5	11.5	8.6
South Asia	568.4	631.9	570.9
Sub-Saharan Africa	204.9	330.0	386.0
Total	1,937.8	1,910.3	1,289.0
Total excluding China	1.102.8	1,277.6	1,116.0
REGION/PERCENTAGE OF POPULATION			
East Asia and Pacific	77.2	50.7	14.3
China	84.0	53.7	13.1
Eastern Europe and Central Asia	1.9	2.9	0.5
Latin America and Caribbean	11.9	11.4	6.5
Middle East and North Africa	9.6	4.8	2.7
South Asia	61.1	51.7	36.0
Sub-Saharan Africa	51.5	59.4	47.5
Total	52.2	40.9	22.4
Total excluding China	40.5	36.6	25.2

Source: World Bank (2012, February).

little dip in 1980) when inequalities, as measured as the ratio of the top twenty countries to the bottom twenty countries, declined a little.

A different and more direct method of measuring changes in poverty around the world is to measure the change in the number of poor *people*. There are two ways of doing this, one utilizing national accounts data and the other using data from national surveys. Table 4 gives the number of people and the proportion of the total population who lived on less than $1.25 in 2005 prices, used by the World Bank as a measure of poverty in various regions and countries of the world in 1981, 1993, and 2008 (the last year for which data were available).

The top portion of Table 4 shows that the total number of poor people in all developing countries declined from 1,937.8 million in 1981 to 1,289.0 million in 2008. As a percentage of the total population of developing countries, the number of poor people declined from 52.2 in 1981 to 22.4 in 2008. Thus, according to this data, there was a dramatic decline in the number and proportion of poor people in the developing world during the most recent period of rapid globalization (1981 to 2008).

Table 4 also shows that from 1981 to 2008, the number of poor declined by 662.1 million in China, 6.0 million in Eastern Europe and Central Asia, 6.5 million in Latin America and the Caribbean, and 7.9 million in the Middle East and North Africa, but it increased by 2.5 million in South Asia and a staggering 181.1 million in Sub-Saharan Africa. As a percentage of the total population (which increased everywhere), however, it declined in every region. The decline was most dramatic in China, where it went from 84.0 percent in 1981 to 13.1 percent in 2008.

For the entire developing world, the same statistic declined from 52.2 percent in 1981 to 22.4 percent in 2008 (but this reflects mostly the sharp decline in China). Despite the general decline in the *percentage* of

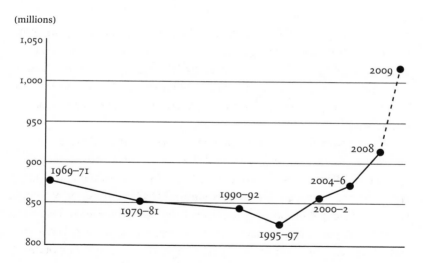

Figure 1. The Number of Hungry People in the World, 1969–71 to 2010 (in millions)

Note: The percentage for 2009 is an estimate.

Source: IMF (March 2010), 40.

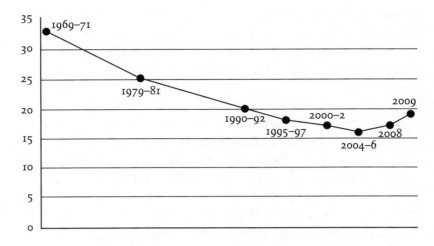

Figure 2. The Percentage of Undernourished People in the World, 1969–71 to 2009 (in millions)

Note: The percentage for 2009 is an estimate.

Source: IMF (March 2010), 40.

very poor people in the world during the past three decades, the number of people suffering hunger in the world has sharply increased from 1995–97 to 2009 (see Figure 1) and so has the percentage of undernourished people from 2004–6 to 2009 (see Figure 2). Thus the great need for economic growth and humanitarian assistance to the poorest countries.

We can therefore arrive at the general conclusion that relative poverty seems to have increased around the world when measured by average national incomes across nations. Looking at individuals rather than nations as a whole, however, we find that the number of people who live in extreme poverty (defined as those who live on less than $1.25 per day in terms of 2005 prices) decreased significantly over the past three decades of rapid globalization, with the exceptions of South Asia and, especially, Sub-Saharan Africa, and with most of the decline occurring in China. As a percentage of the total population (which grew fast in every region), however, it declined almost everywhere, but dramatically only in China. Despite this, the number of hungry people and the percentage of undernourished people in the world increased. The challenge for the world is how to help the poorest nations benefit from globalization, to stimulate their growth over time, and to provide sufficient humanitarian assistance in the meantime to eliminate hunger and undernourishment now.

The Human Development Index (HDI) and World Poverty

There is, of course, another method of measuring the standard of living and poverty in a nation, and that is by HDI, which is calculated annually by the United Nations. This method is a broader, and to some extent a better, measure of the standard of living of a nation because it takes into consideration not only the level of per capita income but also other important conditions of human well-being. The overall HDI is calculated as the average of three indices, the real PPP per capita income, the life expectancy at birth, and the mean years of schooling in the nation, with the last two measures used as catch-alls and proxies for all the other aspects of human well-being besides per capita income. The HDI shows that the difference in the standard of living between rich and poor countries is much smaller than their differences in real per capita incomes and that this difference has declined very much during the past three decades.

Table 5 gives the HDI indices for various HDI groups of countries and regions in 1980, 1990, 2000, and 2011. From the table we see that (1) the HDI index increased for all groups of countries and regions from 1980 to 2011; (2) the index for the very high HDI countries, as a group, was 2.66 times higher than that for the least developed nations in 1980 (much less than the difference in per capita incomes shown in Table 3); and (3) the index of the very high HDI countries was 2.03 times higher than that for the least developed in 2011 (again, much less than in per capita incomes). Future increases in the standard of living of poor nations, however, will very likely depend even more than in the past on increases in real per capita incomes after the basics of life have been provided. After all, health and education are very costly.

Table 5. HDI for Various Groups of Nations, Various Regions, and Least Developed Nations, 1980, 1990, 2000, and 2011

HDI GROUPS	1980	1990	2000	2011
Very high	0.766	0.810	0.858	0.889
High	0.614	0.648	0.687	0.741
Medium	0.420	0.480	0.548	0.630
Low	0.316	0.347	0.383	0.456
Arab states	0.444	0.516	0.578	0.641
HDI REGIONS				
East Asia and Pacific	0.428	0.498	0.581	0.671
Europe and Central Asia	0.644	0.680	0.695	0.751
Latin America and Caribbean	0.582	0.624	0.680	0.731
South Asia	0.356	0.418	0.468	0.548
Sub-Saharan Africa	0.365	0.383	0.401	0.463
Least developed countries	0.288	0.320	0.363	0.439
World	0.558	0.594	0.634	0.682

Source: World Bank (2011a).

The Millennium Development Goals (MDGs) and Targets

In trying to overcome poverty and hunger in the world, the World Bank sponsored the MDGs in 2000, which were signed by 189 countries. The MDGs propose a program for rich countries to help the poorest developing countries stimulate growth, reduce poverty, and promote sustainable development. They specify a set of eight objectives incorporating specific targets for reducing income poverty, tackling other sources of human deprivation, and promoting sustainable development by 2015. These are: (1) halve extreme poverty and hunger relative to 1990; (2) achieve universal primary education; (3) promote gender equality and empower women; (4) reduce child mortality; (5) improve maternal health; (6) combat HIV/AIDS, malaria, and other diseases; (7) ensure environmental sustainability; and (8) establish a global partnership for development (see Table 8 in the Appendix for details of each goal).

By 2009, some of the MDGs scheduled to be reached by 2015 had already been attained, others were within reach, while some were lagging. Goal 1 (halving the percentage of people living in extreme poverty and suffering hunger) had been completely or almost completely achieved (see Figure 4 in the Appendix). Goal 3 (promoting gender equality in primary and secondary education) had been achieved and so was the part of goal 7 that aimed at providing access to safe drinking water. Goal 2 (achieving universal primary school education) was within reach, but not the part of goal 7 that deals with achieving basic sanitation. Lagging were the efforts to achieve goal 4 (cutting the mortality rate of children under the age of five) and especially goal 5 (cutting the maternal mortality rate). These are the areas crying out for greater humanitarian assistance.

Globalization, Poverty, and Governance

In general, globalization greatly benefited the people and the nations that globalized. Almost invariably, the nations with the largest percentage of the population living in extreme poverty, and in which poverty has fallen only a little or not at all, are the nations that did not or could globalize. As pointed out earlier, their poverty is due primarily to internal causes (wars, internal strife, corruption, natural disasters, and the HIV virus). What globalization can be blamed for is its bypassing of some of the poorest countries in the world, leaving millions of children starving and hundreds of millions of people in deep poverty.

Globalization itself is devoid of any ethical content. It only increases efficiency for those people and for those nations that take advantage of it. But economic efficiency cannot and should not be everything. There are important social, political, ethical, and health aspects that cannot be left exclusively to the market. The world can hardly be peaceful with millions of people facing stark poverty, starvation, and hopelessness. But these crucial problems facing the world today would not be solved by slowing down the process of globalization.

What is required to solve or at least greatly reduce the problem of world poverty is the reformation of the entire international economic and financial system so as to spread the benefits of globalization more evenly around the world without leaving out the poorest countries and the poorest people. This can be accomplished by canceling the international debts of the poorest countries, sharply increasing foreign aid (which is now only about 0.21 percent of the GDP of rich countries), and greatly opening up the markets of rich countries to exports from the poorest countries.

The promises made by the rich countries at the Monterrey Conference in March of 2002 to increase foreign aid by 50 percent and to open their markets to the exports from the poorest lands were not only inadequate; they have also not been implemented. And with the deepest financial and economic crisis that the world has experienced since the end of World War II, poverty in the poorest nations of the world reversed its downward trend and has again increased. Nothing less than the complete reform of the international economic and monetary system is required.

In short, the world faces a problem of governance. The poorest nations and the poorest people are simply not franchised. They have very

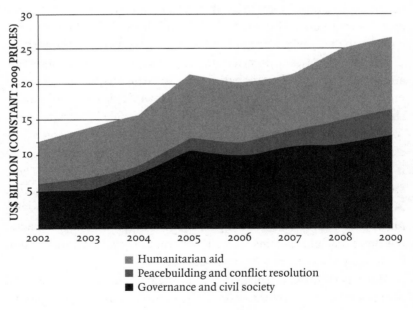

Figure 3. Amount of Various Forms of Aid Spending, 2002–9
Source: UN (2011b), 76.

Table 6. The Top Ten Humanitarian Aid Donors and Recipients in 2009

DONOR	AMOUNT (U.S.$)	RECIPIENT	AMOUNT (U.S.$)
United States	4.4 billion	Sudan	1.4 billion
EU institutions	1.6 billion	Palestine/OPT	1.3 billion
United Kingdom	1.0 billion	Ethiopia	692 million
Germany	727 million	Afghanistan	634 million
Spain	632 million	Somalia	573 million
Sweden	573 million	DRC	567 million
Netherlands	508 million	Pakistan	486 million
France	406 million	Iraq	468 million
Canada	396 million	Kenya	400 million
Norway	375 million	Zimbabwe	393 million

Source: United Nations (2011b), 5.

little say on matters of international economics and finance of great relevance to them. They can only appeal to the humanitarian benevolence of the rich countries. The hope is that with the expansion of the G7 to the G20 (which includes the twelve largest developing countries), the international economic system can be reformed to ensure that the poorest countries and the poorest people of the world also benefit from globalization and that poverty is greatly reduced. It would be truly sad if the selfishness of the G7 were to be replaced by the greed of the G20, if the G20 were to pursue reforms in the management of the world economy to promote primarily their self-interest and abandon the poorest countries to their dismal fate.

Humanitarian Assistance

As we have seen above, there is still a great deal of extreme poverty in the world today. This, together with the needs arising from natural and man-made disasters, results in a great demand for humanitarian assistance to alleviate deep human suffering and despair. Over the past decade, international governments have spent about $90 billion on humanitarian assistance, of which $12.4 billion was spent in 2010. Figure 3 shows the amount and growth of spending on humanitarian aid,

Table 7. Distribution of Humanitarian Assistance Expenditures, 2005–9 (%)

RECIPIENT	NATURAL RELIEF ASSISTANCE	EMERGENCY FOOD AID	RELIEF COORDINATION AND SUPPORT	RECONSTRUCTION RELIEF AND REHABILITATION	DISASTER PREVENTION AND PREPAREDNESS
Afghanistan	29.7	24.9	4.1	40.8	0.5
Ethiopia	17.5	80.5	1.2	0.2	0.6
Haiti	39.4	24.3	3.2	28.2	5.0
Iraq	68.8	2.8	2.1	24.1	2.2
Pakistan	66.3	11.5	3.0	18.3	0.9
Palestine/OPT	69.8	17.3	5.1	7.6	0.1
Sudan	43.4	49.2	2.4	4.9	0.1

Source: United Nations (2011b), 31.

peace-building and conflict resolution, and government and civil society from 2002 to 2009. From the figure we see that all types of aid have increased during 2002–9, but needs far outstripped the aid given. Aid spending often covers no more than about two-thirds of aid needs.

Table 6 shows the top-ten humanitarian aid donors and the top-ten humanitarian aid recipients. As we can see from the table, the United States is the top humanitarian aid donor (and it has been so consistently over the past ten years, providing a total of $31 billion), while Sudan has been the top humanitarian aid recipient over the whole period (it was the leading recipient from 2005 to 2010). This only points to the fact that humanitarian aid is largely long-term in nature, with almost 70 percent going to long-term affected countries and the rest going to disaster relief. Table 7 shows the distribution of humanitarian aid to various specific uses in seven countries over the 2005–9 period.

Conclusions

This chapter examined humanitarian assistance to populations afflicted by major natural and man-made disasters in the broader context of the evolution of world poverty in our rapidly globalizing world. Natural and man-made disasters are generally more common in poor countries than in rich countries, and poor countries are less prepared and able to deal with them than rich countries. Thus the great need for humanitarian assistance to reduce human suffering and despair. A great deal of humanitarian aid is needed for long-term help to relieve chronic poverty, hunger, and malnutrition, and for curing persistent widespread diseases.

The major causes of poverty in the least-developed countries are internal (wars, internal strife, corruption, natural and man-made disasters, and HIV) rather than globalization. In fact, the poorest countries are the ones that have not or could not globalize. What globalization can be accused of is not having permitted the poorest countries to also globalize and share in the great benefits resulting from it.

The powerful force to reduce poverty in the world is economic growth and (as the Commission on Growth and Development's *Growth*

Report indicated) globalization and international competitiveness are essential characteristics of a high-growth strategy.

Although a great deal of humanitarian aid is now needed, the rapid growth of the least developed countries would go a long way in reducing its need in the future. For this to occur, however, rich countries and the large and rapidly growing emerging market economies (i.e., the G20) must increase developmental aid to the poorest countries, cancel foreign debts, open their markets more widely to the products of the poorest countries and, most importantly, change the governance of the world economy by empowering poor countries and poor people. It is in this context that the present need for humanitarian aid is best examined. More humanitarian aid—absolutely. More help to develop and grow rapidly so as to reduce poverty and increase self-reliance—a must.

Further Reading

Barro, Robert J., and Xavier Sala-I-Martin. 2004. *Economic Growth*. 2nd ed. Cambridge, MA: MIT Press.

Bhagwati, Jagdish. 2004. *In Defense of Globalization*. New York: Oxford University Press.

Bhalla, Surjit S. 2002. *Imagine There's No Country*. Washington, DC: Institute for International Economics.

Chen, Shaohua, and Martin Ravallion. 2010. "The Developing World Is Poorer than We Thought, But No Less Successful in the Fight against Poverty." *The Quarterly Journal of Economics* (May): 315–47.

———. 2012. "Why Don't We See Poverty Convergence?" *American Economic Review* (February): 504–23.

Commission on Growth and Development. 2008. *The Growth Report: Strategies for Sustained Growth and Inclusive Development*. Washington, DC: World Bank.

Dollar, David, and Aron Kraay. 2001. "Growth Is Good for the Poor." *Policy Research Working Paper No. 2587*. Washington DC: World Bank.

———. 2004. "Trade, Growth and Poverty." *The Economic Journal* (February): 22–49.

Grilli, Enzo, and Dominick Salvatore. 1994. *Economic Development*. Westport, CT: Greenwood Press.

International Monetary Fund (IMF). 2010. "Regaining Momentum." *Finance and Development* 47: 6–10.

———. 2012. *World Economic Outlook*. Washington, DC: IMF.

Kraay, Aart, and Claudio Raddatz. 2007. "Poverty Traps, Aid, and Growth." *Journal of Development Economics* (March): 315–47.

Pritchett, Lant. 1997. "Divergence, Big Time." *Journal of Economic Perspectives* 3: 3–17.

Salvatore, Dominick. 1993. *Protectionism and World Welfare*. New York: Cambridge University Press.

———. 2010. "Globalization, International Competitiveness, and Growth." *Journal of International Commerce, Economics and Policy* (April): 21–32.

———. 2012. "Trade Policy and Internationalization." Ch 11 in *Knowledge Innovation and Internationalization*, ed. P. Morone (forthcoming from Routledge).

Stern, Nicholas. 2002. *A Strategy for Development*. Washington, DC: World Bank.

Stiglitz, Joseph. 2002. *Globalization and Its Discontents*. New York: Norton & Company.

United Nations (UN). 2011a. *Human Development Report*. New York: UN.

———. 2011b. *GHA Report 2011*. New York: UN.

World Bank. 2002. *Globalization, Growth and Poverty: Building an Inclusive World Economy*. New York: Oxford University Press.

———. 2011a. *The Changing Wealth of Nations*. Washington, DC: World Bank.

———. 2011b. *Multipolarity: The New Global Economy*. Washington, DC: World Bank.

———. 2012, February. "Update of World Bank's Estimates of Consumption Poverty in the Developing World." Washington DC: World Bank. Available from http://siteresources.worldbank.org/INTPOVCALNET/Resources/Global_Poverty_Update_2012_02-29-12.pdf.

———. 2012a. *World Development Indicators*. Washington, DC: World Bank.

———. 2012b. *World Development Report*. Washington, DC: World Bank.

World Commission on the Social Dimension of Globalization. 2004. *A Fair Globalization*. Geneva: ILO.

Appendix

Table 8. Detailed Millennium Development Goals

---

8. Develop a global partnership for development

8a. Develop further an open, rule-based, predictable, nondiscriminatory trading and financial system.

8b. Address the special needs of the least developed countries.

8c. Address the special needs of landlocked developing countries and small island developing states.

8d. Deal comprehensively with the debt problems of developing countries through national and international measures to make debt sustainable in the long term.

8e. In cooperation with pharmaceutical companies, provide access to affordable, essential drugs in developing countries.

8f. In cooperation with the private sector, make available the benefits of new technologies, especially information and communications.

Source: IMF (2010), 7.

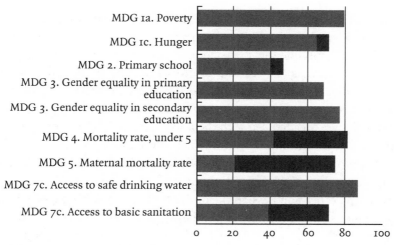

■ Distance to goal achieved by 2009 to be on track for 2015 target

■ Shortfall in progress needed by 2009 to be on track for 2015 target

Figure 4. Progress in Achieving the MDGs by 2010
Source: IMF (2010), 7.

WFP

Organizational Maintenance in Uncertain Times

MASOOD HYDER

There is nothing compelling about the humanitarian imperative. Any nation large or small is free to put its interests before the rescue of its neighbor. Consequently, the volume of assistance raised for emergencies abroad swells and shrinks according to three overlapping sets of calculations: consideration of national interest, perception of threat to some common good, and pure humanitarian concern. When donor countries are preoccupied with their domestic woes, or if they sense no threat to international order, they are likely to display a degree of indifference to the plight of the vulnerable abroad. That is the way of the world, and there is not much the humanitarian community can do about it. On the other hand, when the desire for national advantage and the pursuit of stability coincides with the needs of those at risk, assistance is more freely available. Since the early 1990s, the World Food Programme (WFP) has managed to locate its emergency operations in that exact spot where concern for human suffering coincides with other Western interests. This astute positioning, combined with its operational excellence, has enabled WFP to become the largest emergency response organization in the world. This chapter proposes to review the question of resource constraints and their impact on arrangements for emergency response using the example of this successful agency, including an examination of WFP's survival strategy in an uncertain funding environment, characterized by expanding humanitarian needs in a rapidly transforming political landscape.

The Effect of Economic Constraints on Disaster Response

The WFP example illustrates the tendency of the international community to focus on the most salient disasters, ignoring other large areas of need: people quietly starving in their homes and villages, for example, who, because they do not represent a threat except to themselves, are often left to their own devices, and apparently do not enter the calculus of need. "In our view," noted James Morris, WFP Executive Director at the time (2005), addressing the United Nations (UN) Security Council, "there are few phenomena in modern life as political as humanitarian aid. The world's major donors all make clearly political choices on which humanitarian aid projects to fund."[1]

Every year, WFP assists over 100 million people on average, in eighty countries across the globe. That is a remarkable achievement in itself, but it represents less than 10 percent of the hungry poor, and an even smaller fraction of the total if those who suffer from micronutrient deficiencies are included. In referring to "diminishing resources," we mean a fall in the resources available for disasters considered most risky both politically and in humanitarian terms, directed toward persons who actually represent a small fraction of those in need.

Even within this narrow category of humanitarian need, requirements have gone up, for several reasons. This is first due to the fourfold increase in the occurrence of natural disasters (up from 900 in the 1970s to over 4,000 in the first decade of this century);[2] second, to the global rise in food prices and continuing market volatility, which has resulted in the numbers of the hungry reaching the 1 billion mark, and food aid costing more because of the increase in food and fuel prices.[3] Third, there is an increasing tendency for humanitarian operations to move into the theaters of war which, combined with a certain erosion of acceptance and respect for aid workers, has added enormously to the cost of ensuring their safety. In January 2007, the UN had 210 security professionals in the field, managed by the Department for Safety and Security (DSS), not including security professionals hired by the UN agencies or by the Department of Peacekeeping Operations (DPKO). By

2012 it had 600 field personnel, and was managing 130 staff from the various agencies, funds, and programs. It also deployed over 1,000 staff in the uniformed DSS (the blue-uniformed security at UN Headquarters in New York, Geneva, Vienna, Nairobi, and eight other locations). In addition, the DPKO's civilian and security staff numbers had grown to 3,000, comprised of both international and locally recruited staff.[4] Fourth, aid is increasingly being used as a tool of military policy, to stabilize governments and win over populations. This takes up an ever-increasing proportion of humanitarian and development budgets, diverts assistance from peaceful regions to insurgency-affected areas, and compromises the essential neutrality of aid.[5]

It is true that humanitarian *requirements* have gone up but there is also a remarkable rise in humanitarian budgets, at least until 2010, after which year the detailed reports are not yet in. Resources of the international humanitarian enterprise have gone up from $2 billion in 2000 to $7 billion in 2007, reaching $16.7 billion in 2012. Indeed, this growing capacity of the UN agencies and its NGO partners has itself created an expectation of response, which in turn has the effect of pushing requirements upwards. It is not surprising, therefore, that in reviewing the results of its consolidated appeal for major emergencies in 2010, the Office for the Coordination of Humanitarian Affairs (OCHA) noted both a record level of funding at $6.6 billion and a slight fall in the percentage of requirements met, at 59 percent (as against 64 percent in 2009, or 55 percent in 2005).[6]

There is little conclusive evidence of a decline in humanitarian assistance for another reason. Take the case of WFP. Since it is voluntarily funded, it is difficult to predict the size of contributions in the absence of prior commitment. And since humanitarian assistance is responsive to disasters, an emergency budget may seem precarious until some disaster prompts governments to give. The WFP budget for 2007 was $2.7 billion and went up to $5 billion in 2008 when governments became aware of the magnitude of the food crisis.[7] Humanitarian assistance may be unpredictable, but it is clearly responsive to need. This suggests that it is not the state of budgets but *capacity to respond* that is perhaps a better, though indirect, indicator of preparedness. If WFP ran down its ability to deal with disasters, cutting down its capacity to

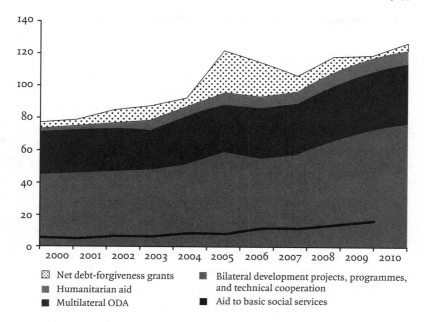

Figure 1. Main Components of Official Development Assistance (ODA) for Development Assistance Committee (DAC) Members, 2000–10 (billions of 2009 dollars)

Source: Organization for Economic Cooperation and Development/Development Assistance Committee (OECD/DAC) data.

deal with emergencies before donor funding arrived, and no longer qualified for loans from the Central Emergency Response Fund (CERF); if it gave up the Brindisi warehouse facility and generally ran down its readiness, then that would indicate that humanitarian assistance was indeed in decline. This has not happened.

To summarize: humanitarian budgets have risen dramatically in the first decade of this century; any dips more recently certainly do not push them back to turn-of-century levels. Humanitarian funding is responsive to disasters and underfunded budgets can fill up quickly following a disaster. Any strain on funding does not appear to have affected preparedness. Western donors are still capable of responding to humanitarian need abroad despite their economic problems. The aid budget represents a small fraction of government revenue. In 2009, out of U.S. government revenues of $4,352 billion, total aid was $29 billion, of which humanitarian assistance accounted for $4.4 billion, that is, 0.001 percent or one thousandth of government revenue.[8] Development aid budgets are shrinking due to economic constraints, but that is less true of humanitarian funding because the latter responds more directly to changes in the political climate. In view of these considerations, the issue of declining budgets becomes somewhat less alarming.

Low funding during a recession is worrying but not grave; recessions end, and funding may rebound. Of greater concern is the use of humanitarian assistance in support of military objectives. There can be other radical shifts in the methods of attending to the arrangements of society that would denote a more permanent change. For example, the humanitarian enterprise may fall out of favor with its Western backers, who might turn to other more amenable instruments of policy; or, the emerging powers such as China, India, Brazil, Russia, and others might choose not to support it. These eventualities pose a threat to the very survival of the humanitarian enterprise.[9]

Organizational Maintenance in Uncertain Times

In an uncertain funding environment, with expanding humanitarian needs and a rapidly changing aid scene, what is WFP's strategy? Like all organizations, it too must attract the resources necessary to survive and to achieve its goals. The basic objective of all bureaucracies (to use James Q. Wilson's phrase) is "organizational maintenance."[10] The scramble for resources, as much as its mandate, determines an organization's behavior. In order to accomplish its goals, WFP offers incentives, notably its operational expertise, and its access to those in need. These characteristic incentives both shape WFP strategy and constrain its actions.

Maintaining Support and Managing Constraints

The main challenges for WFP concern building and maintaining support, and managing constraints. This involves WFP in a delicate balancing act: if its goals are too ambitious or idealistic it risks the indifference of its traditional donors; if too pragmatic or conservative, it risks alienating the recipient countries. The balancing act is in evidence in a number of crucial strategic decisions that determine how well WFP's goals can be reached, especially at times when it is threatened with resource constraints. Using this model, it is proposed to examine some areas of policy where funding considerations are involved.

KEEPING LEAN AND MEAN

WFP depends entirely on voluntary funding, a form of support that could be easily turned off if donors are not satisfied with its performance. As a consequence, WFP runs a tight operation, keeping administrative and operational costs as low as possible. From time to time it has to check the tendency for expenditures to rise. High food prices from 2007 onwards resulted in more money being spent on purchases and services. Overheads charged by WFP increased, and some of that income went into the recruitment of additional staff, whose numbers grew. As a result WFP is in a position to shed some fat if it wishes, given that it currently has high numbers of senior staff. Generally speaking, UN agencies are not particularly transparent, but it pays to be accountable to donors, and this will be an easy win for the organization. On the other hand, the decision to hold on to additional emergency response capacity in anticipation of the next disaster (as discussed earlier) is a calculated risk at best. Not all funding decisions are so entirely in the hands of WEP, as the next example concerning its efforts to widen the pool of donors demonstrates.

GETTING THE NONTRADITIONAL DONORS ON BOARD

It is often overlooked that food is a major component in humanitarian operations. If the donor base is to be widened in terms of food resources, it is necessary to find ways of bringing in the so-called nontraditional food donors. In September 2001, the Indian government wrote to a number of the least-developed, food-deficit countries, offering them wheat, free of charge, if they would bear the cost of transportation. There had been a series of bumper harvests that had increased India's strategic grain stocks well beyond requirements. The government's guarantee to farmers that it would support wheat prices had obliged it to purchase several million tons of wheat.[11] There is no record available of how many takers the Government of India found for its generous offer. A little later, India donated a million tons of wheat to WFP for the Afghanistan program.

India, long reliant on food imports and PL-480 grants, was finally in a position to give back. It was in this spirit that the Indian delegation announced its offer at WFP's Executive Board.[12] But its triumph turned to consternation when some European members expressed their reservations about India's offer, noting that it should look to its own poor (recalling E.H. Carr's observation that diplomats cloak the interests of their country in the language of universal justice). The Indian delegate responded with barely suppressed anger. Why could India not give, he asked, when it had been producing surpluses of 10–20 million tons of grain annually? Since when, he demanded, had WFP become a rich man's club?

Of course, other major donors rose in support of India's gesture. But to this day, no procedure put in place by WFP has succeeded in overcoming the hesitations first hinted at during that Executive Board meeting. There are four cost components to any transaction involving food aid: purchase price of cereal, sea freight, transportation inside recipient country, and administrative costs of monitoring and supervision. Of these, the price of cereals is two-thirds of the total. Therefore, if the food is available gratis, then total cost falls dramatically. The Indian offer was not accompanied by the usual cash element that traditional donors were used to providing. In order to facilitate food-only donations, WFP had devised a procedure, termed "twinning," whereby food donations such as India's could be matched with cash donations from other cash donors. This arrangement has worked sporadically, but there is no rule on the books that obliges WFP to look for free food donations first. It took WFP several years to gradually accept the million-ton donation from India, in small tranches, as and when it could arrange the associated costs.

Normally donor countries look closely at expenditures and come down hard on missed opportunities to make their taxpayers' contribution stretch further. In this case, the benefits are so obvious that it is tempting to ask why cash donors among the traditional supporters of WFP do not insist that it look for free cereal donation and use their cash for covering administration and transportation costs.

On their side, the nontraditional donors have not shown much enthusiasm either. Aid from non–Organization for Economic Co-operation and Development (OECD) members has grown dramatically, up from $4 billion in 2005 to $12 billion in 2008,[13] but it has stayed outside the Western OECD Development Assistance Committee (DAC) system. The BRICs (Brazil, Russia, India, and China) in particular seem to be developing their own style of aid largely focusing on bilateral assistance to neighboring countries, and, while employing the rhetoric of South–South cooperation, using aid as a means of supporting their commercial interests. There are signs since 2011 that the BRICs are beginning to give more through multilateral channels, but it remains to be seen how far they adopt the policies of Western donors, or how warmly they are welcomed into Western institutions.

THE MUSLIM WORLD AS POTENTIAL DONOR

Muslim countries constitute a potential nontraditional donor group for two reasons: 1) because the majority of those receiving humanitarian assistance worldwide are Muslim; and 2) because Islam has well-developed concepts of—and elaborate arrangements for—charitable giving. These reasons constitute strong arguments for assuming that the Muslim states would be valuable participants in the humanitarian enterprise and generous donors to its programs. And yet, the relationship is distant though friendly, and marked by a certain lack of interest on either side.

Muslim beneficiaries appear to predominate in all categories of aid: emergency, development, and refugee operations. Humanitarian agencies do not keep records of recipients differentiated by religion. Using Organisation of Islamic Cooperation (OIC) membership as a proxy indicator, it is estimated that about half of WFP beneficiaries hail from Muslim countries.[14] Thus, even after allowing for overlapping clientele between WFP and other humanitarian agencies, direct recipients of humanitarian assistance have easily numbered over 50 million Muslims at any given time over the past ten years.[15] Of course not all recipients from OIC countries are Muslim, but that discrepancy is more than made up for by the existence of significant Muslim minorities in non-OIC states. Given the strained relationship between the West and the Muslim world, this large-scale and beneficent contact is remarkable—and unremarked.

Traditional Muslim concepts of charity (*zakat*, *sadaqa*, and *waqf*) and the contemporary idea of humanitarian assistance are close but not identical, and perhaps it is one of those cases where small differences ensure separation. There is a very large literature on Islamic giving covering the three concepts.[16] *Zakat* is obligatory and payable only to Muslim beneficiaries who are specified in the Qur'an (Sura 9, v. 60), and whose status has been much discussed by Muslim jurists. *Zakat* therefore does not really qualify as being the equivalent of humanitarian aid in modern terms. *Sadaqa*, especially one particular kind designated as *sadaqat al-tatawwu'* (alms of spontaneity) is voluntary and can be given to Muslim and non-Muslim alike without further specification of their status or need. This type of *sadaqa* is therefore more akin to humanitarian aid in modern terms. *Waqf* does not come into the picture because it involves endowment of property and the establishment of foundations, and there is no evidence of *waqf* income from property endowments going as a voluntary contribution to international agencies.

There has been a great deal of discussion among jurists about how these terms, in particular *zakat*, should be treated in a modern context, and different Muslim countries have adopted different strategies. The interface between the Muslim concepts of *sadaqa*, *zakat*, *waqf*, and humanitarian assistance remains largely unexplored. Whatever the points of difference, they seem to have little impact on humanitarian operations in Muslim countries. OIC members welcome humanitarian agencies to their meetings as observers, have passed helpful resolutions (for example expressing appreciation of the UN High Commissioner for Refugees' work), and in general have good relations with international humanitarian agencies, both as contributors and as recipients. Thus there seems to be broad agreement on the underlying purposes.

There are no reliable figures for philanthropic giving in Muslim communities. One source estimated them to be in the range of $250 billion to $1 trillion annually.[17] This seems rather high. Some *waqf* endowments are indeed very rich, but most are inefficiently managed, usually by government bureaucrats. They are at varying stages of reform in different countries, from India to Libya, but nowhere seem to be organized along business lines. Apparently, neither the World Bank nor the UN Development Agencies have so far proposed a project designed to improve *waqf* income.

The Alterman study proposes that the United States consider utilizing Islamic charitable organizations, and not confine itself to Western NGOs as a channel of assistance, although if, as the study states, Muslims have $250 billion to $1 trillion available through their own sources, it is not clear why they would be interested in the relatively modest sums the West could supply.

Muslim governments are also to blame for accepting the status quo and for not adopting a policy of increasing their influence on assistance agencies by taking a far more active role as donors, partners, and suppliers of qualified staff. In this way the Arab Gulf states who could do so much more have always treated UN agencies as western channels, and have provided only symbolic support to them. There have been sporadic donations, some of them very large (such as the $500 million donation to WFP in 2008 during the food crisis), but nothing as consistent as their promotion of education in Afghanistan, Pakistan, and elsewhere around the world, which represents one of their main channels of foreign assistance.

BALANCING HUNGER AND SECURITY ISSUES

There is a temptation to link hunger with security, especially given that political mobilization for hunger is an uphill task.[18] In a general sense, there is certainly a link between hunger and security: crop failures have a major impact on a country's economy, and on its perception of strategic self-sufficiency. A state may feel insecure if its strategic stocks of food run low, and drought could cause a people to move, with unpredictable consequences for the stability of the region as a whole.

Mainline economic analysis seems to concur. Jeffrey Sachs, for instance, observes that economic failure can lead to state failure. By not meeting basic needs of the people, failed states can become the seedbeds of violence and terror. Therefore the question of ending poverty, hunger, and disease must be taken seriously.[19] Such analyses point to a dangerous trend, not to an imminent threat. They look at root causes and propose fundamental economic changes over time.[20]

There are other observers who appear to suggest that a more direct link exists between hunger and violence, creating an imminent threat. The argument verges on the alarmist. It ignores the fact, for instance, that the world has a billion hungry but peaceful people. On June 23, 2005, President Obasanjo of Nigeria wrote an op-ed in the British newspaper the *Guardian*, in which he stated that "a hungry person is an angry and dangerous person." His comment was quoted with approval back and forth a week later by several participants at hearings at the UN Security Council on "Africa's food crises as a threat to peace and security," including the main speaker, the executive director of the WFP.[21] The hearings were unusual in that the Security Council, exceptionally, abandoned its customary understanding that hunger was a social and economic issue (and therefore of interest to the UN Economic and Social Council [ECOSOC]) to temporarily embrace the idea that it might pose a threat to peace and security.

The UN's experience with the hungry poor in Asia and Africa conveys a different impression altogether. WFP usually assists people whose sources of food have diminished catastrophically, causing them to suffer serious debilitation if not outright starvation. In that condition they are hardly likely to take up arms. But it is not just their weakened condition that constrains them. In traditional societies, hunger and disease are regarded as providential visitations against which it is useless to struggle. Others, with modern sensibilities, might protest if they were short of food, but this is not the case with the rural poor, who bear their suffering with great fortitude, in silence and dignity. This is not to deny the occurrence of bread riots, but they are an urban phenomenon. They are provoked by sudden price rises (or "price spikes") which alarm and even upset governments, as seen in 2008. The point is that the threat to order comes from the politically aware urban masses, still in possession of sufficient energy to protest. But treating a hungry person as an angry person runs the risk of ignoring humanitarian principles and transforming, in effect, an obligation to help into a necessity to placate.

Poverty, hunger, peace, and security are linked in many ways but it is too simplistic to derive direct causal links between them. Removing poverty removes a long-term risk to political and economic stability. This is different from stating that the poor are dangerous, or adopting that as a basis of action. The short-term concern with price spikes and their consequences is justified so long as it is recognized that it derives from political considerations that have more to do with the stability of governments than with the welfare of people.

Just as access to oil has influenced foreign policies, food security too seems to have infiltrated the national security domain. WFP has carefully skirted the issue, sometimes coming close to making the linkage. "Without food," declared Josette Sheeran, executive director of WFP, in 2010, "people do one of three things: revolt, migrate, or starve."[22] However, its projects and operations continue to be proposed in humanitarian, not security terms. On the other hand, despite its profound institutional knowledge of poverty and hunger issues, it has stayed outside the hunger-security debate.

RAISING FUNDS DURING THE FOOD CRISIS OF 2008

The same impression of maintaining a sense of its own priorities was evident in WFP's role in the 2008 food crisis. While playing its part in the High-Level Task Force (HLTF) set up by the Secretary-General to deal with the crisis, WFP continued its own advocacy for the hungry, aimed at three urgent tasks: raising additional funds to meet higher costs affecting its approved portfolio of projects for 2008; expanding its operations in order to cover the needs of the newly hungry; and coping with large new emergencies resulting from natural disasters. WFP met all three objectives. Given that it fully relies on voluntary donations, it was an extraordinary achievement, not only in fundraising but also in terms of operational efficiency and effective communication.

In practical terms, WFP's achievements in 2008 owed little directly to the efforts of the HLTF. Most of the funds were raised before the publication of the Comprehensive Framework for Action (CFA) under the direction of the HLTF.[23] True, the UN Secretary-General and the World Bank President went out of their way to appeal on behalf of WFP, but this was largely done outside the HLTF context. WFP's successful fundraising did not stem from the coordination mechanisms that were created.

It is difficult to say if the CFA's recommendations helped the HLTF members in any practical way, although the symbolism was powerful: working together, the UN system, including the Bretton Woods Institutions (BWIs), had quickly produced an excellent document. But the CFA itself and the goodwill generated did very little in 2008 to help directly, for example, smallholder farmers of Africa (a major recommendation of the CFA). The planting season came and went without much notice being taken of their plight. This was the great failure of 2008, which went largely unnoticed by the media. Direct results are very difficult to measure if the objectives are coordination and enhancing coherence. It is notable how UN agencies cooperate in joint endeavors without losing their sense of a separate identity and continue to pursue their individual priorities.

"ONE UN" AS POTENTIALLY INHIBITING HUMANITARIAN ACTION

In Libya, much is expected of the UN, which has come to figure as the guarantor of transition and is trusted by Libyans more than their bilateral benefactors. The UN's integrated mission not only attempts to bring together the different agencies, funds, programs, and departments of the UN system, but also coordinates with major international entities that deal directly with the Libyan authorities while collaborating with the UN, notably the BWIs and the European Union. This integrated approach not only coordinates powerful entities but also attempts to organize three sets of disparate actions: humanitarian, developmental, and political. The three responses are by their very nature divergent, operating on different timescales with different funding sources, and answerable to different authorities. More importantly, they answer the question "How is stabilization best achieved?" differently. This last calls for a difficult balancing act between the pursuit of order and social justice.

The functionalist approach (that governs most agencies, funds, and programs) focuses directly on economic, social, technical, and humanitarian matters, believing these "nonpolitical" objectives to be a prerequisite for establishing durable peace and long-term stability. The political approach puts greater emphasis on measures designed to ensure order and stability in the short run. Historically, the UN system, by keeping these priorities separate, had tacitly acknowledged that the two could be better served by working side by side. While integrating UN activities at country level makes sense in terms of good management, there is the risk that in promoting a unified approach at country level the functionalist principle would be overwhelmed by peace and security initiatives. Here then is another way in which, potentially, the scope of humanitarian action can be restricted.

Conclusions

There is an endless dialectic between idealism and realism. In the end it is not humanitarian theory that creates practice; it is practice that establishes the scope for humanitarian theory and defines the limits of humanitarian action. "There is no greater barrier to clear political thinking," wrote E.H. Carr in *The Twenty Years' Crisis*, "than failure to distinguish between ideals, which are utopian, and institutions, which are reality."

Existing in the real world, organizations act as if only the paranoid survive. Funding strains are constantly in evidence whether or not donor economies are thriving. The cases outlined here bring out aspects of this underlying principle of organizational maintenance: that donors' concerns about expenditures must be respected; that an organization may look for new funding sources without alienating the regular donors; that it is not done to openly criticize donor policy even if it comes close to undermining humanitarian principles; that funding should remain an agency's particular concern even while cooperating with other partners. Of course humanitarian action is not restricted by financial constraints alone. The integration of different parts of the

UN system, designed to work with a certain degree of autonomy, may well inhibit humanitarian action too, as in the case of "One UN" arrangements at country level.

The funding preoccupation can act quite insidiously on an organization to weaken its resolve. The fear of opposition by traditional donors can mute dissent and shape the way a subordinate organization reacts, even one as powerful as WFP. While, at the best of times, WFP has nurtured an institutional culture based on the free exchange of ideas and the promotion of initiative and risk-taking, characteristics that have sustained its operational excellence, it can display a different side of its persona when dealing with the donors, becoming understated, careful, and compliant. This change suggests that there might be a rule of anticipated reaction in play in these interactions.

Apart from funding preoccupations, all humanitarian agencies are affected by the shortcomings of the international disaster relief system, some of which have been rehearsed in the course of this chapter. The system is too focused on conflicts, post hoc in its response, investing too little in preparedness, ineffectual at ensuring transition to development, and paternalistic in its approach to recipients. This is a familiar list. What is new is the arrival of the emerging economies on the scene, led by the BRICs, that are able but not willing to join wholeheartedly in the humanitarian enterprise, or put off by the lukewarm reception they have received. What is also new is the securitization of humanitarian action. These are alarming developments because for the present a functioning humanitarian enterprise is needed. But perhaps in the future national capacities will improve, and states will depend less on international assistance. It is considered that Africa, currently the main consumer of humanitarian assistance, is already on the path to rapid economic growth, developing faster than any other region in the world. Foreign direct investment is flowing in at double the rate of aid. In the next couple of decades it may substantially outgrow the need for foreign aid.[24]

What is certain is that the aid environment is changing and there is a need to readapt to the conditions of a new, emerging historical epoch. Otherwise the present arrangements may not survive, and it is difficult to predict what will take their place. "I fear for the future of the shared impulse to which organized humanitarian efforts attempt to give practical meaning. In my judgment, the humanitarian enterprise is living on borrowed time," wrote Larry Minear in 2002.[25] But for all its shortcomings, the humanitarian system has demonstrated that something can be done to alleviate the age-old miseries of famine, war, and disease, and that we need not be passive victims of fate. That might well be its enduring legacy.

This chapter has dealt with WFP's relations with its donors, being primarily concerned with funding issues. Access, involving WFP's relations with recipient countries, and beneficiary issues, involving WFP's accountability to its 100 million clients, also raise fundamental questions that were not considered here.

Disasters—A Nation's Experience in an Economic Recession

RONAN MURPHY

How does a government which is concerned about the plight of poor people caught up in disasters around the world but which has limited resources to help deliver a good product in terms of disaster response and disaster preparedness? That is the question this chapter addresses, using Ireland as an example of a country that is currently facing this dilemma.

The Irish people have shown themselves to be remarkably generous over the years in their response to poor people's needs, especially in Africa. The reasons for this have often been debated. Geopolitical concerns do not feature as they do for some countries. Rather, like the Scandinavian countries, Ireland's approach is primarily founded on an altruistic desire to help.

The example of the country's missionaries—mostly Catholic but with a strong Protestant missionary tradition also—has probably been the single largest factor in shaping the Irish people's attitudes. These missionaries have been meeting the basic needs of the poor, and above all bringing them education, for almost two centuries.

Folk memories of Ireland's Great Famine of the 1840s are also cited. It seems a long time ago, you might say. But the Famine, with over a million deaths and a quarter of the population emigrating, cast a long shadow over Ireland's history and the memory has not gone away. In fact, today there is greater awareness of, and interest in, the Famine, with a national commemoration and a Famine Museum.

This high level of concern for the poor is particularly demonstrated in the Irish people's response to disasters in the developing world. Private donations from the Irish have long been among the largest per head of population—Ethiopia in the 1980s, Somalia and Rwanda in the 1990s, the Indian Ocean tsunami in 2004. Even in recent years, when economic times have turned harsh and people have less to give, Irish people have donated generously to disasters such as Haiti, the Pakistan floods, and the drought in the Horn of Africa.

And not just with money: people have been willing to drop everything to go and help. Doctors and nurses, housing and nutrition experts, emergency personnel and ordinary citizens have left their jobs to assist. Whenever I have visited disaster response efforts, Irish nongovernmental organizations (NGOs) and relief workers have invariably been present. I will come back to the issue of public support because I see it as a key factor.

Ireland's official program of assistance to the developing world began in 1973 and so is almost forty years old. It is delivered through a division of the country's Department of Foreign Affairs, known as Irish Aid.

From the start, the program took the classical form with three main areas of activity: support for the United Nations (UN) funds and bodies, the Bretton Woods Institutions and other multilateral funders; a bilateral program focused on a limited number of countries; and disaster response. Despite having grown significantly in volume over the four decades, Irish Aid's activities today continue to be concentrated on these three areas.

Disaster response has been a central element of the Irish Aid program from the start—indeed it can be said that it predated the setting up of a proper development aid program. This reflects the simple fact—not confined to Ireland—that public engagement with the plight of poor countries is spurred on by the very visible evidence of disasters both natural and man-made.

Ireland's funding for disaster response was at first channeled almost exclusively through multilateral organizations such as the UN humanitarian bodies and the Red Cross. A further feature that emerged over time was cooperation between the Government and Ireland's NGOs, which are numerous and active.

From the 1990s until 2008, as Irish Aid expanded the amount of money allocated by the Government to disaster response increased significantly. This was the so-called Celtic Tiger era when Ireland experienced gross national product growth rates of 6 and 7 percent a year and money for public spending was freely available.

During those prosperous years Ireland seemed, for the first time, about to reach the Holy Grail: the UN target of spending 0.7 percent of gross national income (GNI) on official development assistance. The year 2008 saw a total of €921 million—more than $1 billion—spent on development aid, the equivalent of 0.59 percent of GNI. The projections were that in 2009 expenditure on ODA would reach 0.65 percent of GNI. The amounts spent on disaster response during the good years increased proportionately.

But Ireland has suffered a huge economic reverse. A toxic combination of bad banking practices, weak oversight, and a property bubble caused a crash that turned the country from boom to bust in the space of a few years. November 2008 stands out as a black moment for Ireland when the Government was faced with the likely collapse of its banks and decided to give a blanket guarantee to the system. Within a few months Ireland had no option but to apply to the International Monetary Fund and the European institutions for a bailout.

Since 2008, Ireland has been transformed from being a model for economic growth to one of the most highly indebted countries in the

Table 1. Ireland's Official Development Assistance (ODA) as a Percentage of GNI, 2007–11

	TOTAL ODA (MILLIONS OF EUROS)	% OF GNI
2007	871	0.54
2008	921	0.59
2009	722	0.55
2010	676	0.53
2011 (est.)	655	0.52

Table 2. Ireland's Budget for Disaster Relief, 2007–11

	MILLION EUROS
2007	121
2008	109
2009	68
2010	64
2011 (est.)	66

Note: These figures include the three main humanitarian budget lines managed by Irish Aid's Emergency and Recovery Section: the Emergency Humanitarian Assistance Fund, the Emergency Preparedness, Post-Emergency and Recovery Assistance Fund, and the Rapid Response Initiative.

world. Remarkably, a substantial aid program has managed to survive although, as the figures show in Tables 1 and 2, the overall volume has fallen by a third between 2008 and 2011. The biggest cut—€200 million came in 2009. Since then there have been smaller cuts.

The budget for disaster relief also fell—from a high of €121 million in 2007 to €66 million in 2011.

The fall in volume of the aid budgetary figures underlines the challenges that Irish Aid faces. It is not just the money that has been cut; staffing levels have suffered as the Government makes determined moves to reduce the size of the public service. Yet Ireland's reputation as a donor remains high. It continues to score well in surveys of international aid programs.

In the OECD's most recent assessment, the October 2011 mid-term review of Ireland by the Development Assistance Committee (DAC), the reviewer says that he was "greatly impressed by the expertise, energy and enthusiasm demonstrated by the Irish Aid team, especially in the light of the extremely challenging domestic context in which they are working." He concludes: "I consider that they [Irish Aid] are well placed to respond to the opportunities and to meet the development challenges that lie ahead."[1] Speaking in Dublin this year, the chair of the DAC Brian Atwood said that Ireland scored highest of all DAC member states when quality tests were applied.

An important feature of the post-boom era has been the Government's reiteration of its commitment to continue funding a strong aid program, in spite of the economic problems Ireland faces. In Irish Aid's annual report for 2010 the ministers for foreign affairs and overseas development said:

> We recognize the need to play our part in responding to emergencies and humanitarian crises. We also recognize our obligation to work with poor countries and communities to help them to take control of their destinies and bring about sustainable long term change. The Government is committed to development cooperation as a central part of Ireland's foreign policy. Despite the serious challenges we face at home, we will strive to meet the targets we have agreed for Official Development Assistance.[2]

This sent a clear political signal that, even if Ireland is facing huge economic challenges at home, it would still not be found wanting in its long tradition of helping the poorest.

So how has Ireland set about working effectively with less money available? The overall approach has been to protect the core values and business of the program. Given the magnitude of the funding reductions, it was clear that all of the three main areas of expenditure—bilateral support for long-term development, emergency and recovery relief, and contributions to multilateral organizations—would have to experience cuts. But it was felt that development cooperation with Ireland's program countries and funding to civil society and NGOs were a top priority.

Ireland's long-term partners—East Timor, Ethiopia, Lesotho, Malawi, Mozambique, Tanzania, Uganda, Vietnam, and Zambia—were specially chosen on the grounds of extreme poverty, as well as factors such as relative stability, capacity to absorb aid and a fit with Irish Aid's approach. Commitments had been entered into with these program countries and it was important that these should continue to be honored. In the event, only East Timor saw its Development Cooperation Office closed and, even there, a reduced program of assistance will continue.

Supporting civil society and Ireland's NGOs has been a cornerstone of Ireland's approach. The country stands out as having more NGOs than most developed countries and NGO funding is proportionately higher in Ireland than in any other country. The NGOs are key partners for the delivery of the Government's aid allocations, both for long-term assistance and emergency response. There is close cooperation and synergy between Irish Aid and the NGOs. A program whereby delegated funding is provided on a multiannual basis was begun in the early years of the new millennium and this has proved remarkably successful. So, when the expenditure axe fell, there was agreement on all sides that funding for the NGOs should be maintained insofar as was feasible in the newly constrained situation. The most obvious target for cuts was on the multilateral side.

In the days of growth and wealth when Ireland could support a wide range of development actors, the multilateral organizations benefited. Ireland's contributions to some of the biggest UN funds and bodies were increased substantially, making Ireland a serious player on the multilateral scene. The scale of funding to the UN Development Programme, the United Nations Children's Fund (UNICEF), the UN High Commissioner for Refugees (UNHCR), and the World Food Program (WFP) grew exponentially between 2000 and 2008. Not only these big organizations but smaller bodies such as the UN Population Fund, the Joint UN Program on HIV/AIDS, the UN Relief and Works Agency, the International Fund for Agricultural Development, the World Health Organization (WHO), the Office of the UN High Commissioner for Human Rights (UNCHR), and a host of others under the aegis of the UN benefited. Ireland also made substantial contributions to the International Development Association and joined the Asian Development Bank.

Worthwhile though it would have been to continue to support these organizations, where savings were essential, reductions had to be made. This was not an easy exercise, any more than cutting other areas of expenditure would have been. Support for the UN and its operations in all their forms, is a bulwark of Ireland's foreign policy. Ireland has an excellent record when it comes to pledging (and, more importantly, delivering) financial support to the UN. Ireland also has got a proud record for its UN peacekeeping in the world's trouble spots, most recently through substantial involvement in the peacekeeping missions to Chad and Liberia.

Maintaining Ireland's strong record on disaster relief was seen as highly important. In many ways, disaster relief is the public face of any aid program, the aspect which the public are most interested in. Funding cuts were not as severe here as in the case of the multilateral organizations but the budget did not escape—as mentioned above, it came down significantly, from €121 million in 2007 to €66 million in 2011. It has been a case of making the best of a smaller budget, to make what funding is available stretch as far as possible. In this, Ireland was well placed on a number of fronts. Most important of all: it had a coherent, comprehensive approach to disaster response and preparedness in place.

A lot of thought and planning around disaster response had been going on in Irish Aid over the previous decade. To understand the background it is necessary to go back and consider why these reflections had been taking place about how to respond effectively to disasters and sudden onset emergencies.

The tsunami in the Indian Ocean at Christmas 2004 marked a turning point in Irish Aid's approach. Yet even before that, the issue of how best to react to emergencies, what kind of help was most valuable and who should provide it, were questions that occupied the attention of Irish Aid, just as it did of many donors.

Ireland was one of seventeen donor governments that joined together in Stockholm in 2003 to form the Good Humanitarian Donorship (GHD) initiative. GHD is an informal forum and network that facilitates collective advancement of its principles and good practices. Behind the setting up of GHD lay a sense that international response to disasters could and should be improved. It is an approach that has drawn increasing support over the years—today GHD has thirty-seven countries subscribing to its principles.

Speeches by Irish representatives at donor conferences around that time emphasized the importance of doing the job better: "The challenges we face are not unique. As donors we have garnered valuable experience and lessons . . . Our aim must be to avoid the mistakes of the past and incorporate the lessons learned in a practical way in all our recovery and reconstruction activities. I cannot overemphasise the importance of coordination in all phases of the reconstruction effort."[3]

The 2004 tsunami put these issues to the test. This cataclysmic event, which cost a quarter of a million lives and affected a dozen countries, most importantly Thailand, Indonesia and Sri Lanka, called for all of the international community's skills, capacities and determination. Massive relief operations took place in the regions affected.

Ireland was not found wanting: the Government allocated a total of €20 million while the Irish public donated an astonishing €80 million. But, as well as delivering immediate assistance, there was a feeling that lessons had to be learned. Irish Aid commissioned a series of reports that would shape Ireland's approach to disaster response and preparedness.

Ireland also joined a consortium of donors, known as the Tsunami Evaluation Coalition Consortium or TEC for short. Over forty agencies took part in this evaluation which resulted in one of the most detailed, comprehensive studies to date of a disaster and the international response so far compiled.[4]

One of the most striking findings in all of these reports, and one which all practitioners of disaster response would do well to heed, was the vital importance of local people in disaster response. The studies found that far more casualties are rescued and lives saved by local people than by outsiders. Another, fairly obvious, recommendation from all sides was that better coordination was needed in emergency response.

A specific concern raised in the reports was the multiplicity of organizations funded by Ireland (this was the main fault that the *Value for Money* report identified in an otherwise very favorable verdict on Irish Aid's performance). This certainly reflected my own thinking at the time: the sight of hundreds of tents and cabins of donors in Banda Aceh, each with its separate logo, ought to have been reassuring since it reflected people's generous instincts. Instead I found it disquieting that so many different actors were involved in the relief effort.

A fourth concern that arose was the importance of moving swiftly from disaster relief to the recovery phase. The risk of temporary shelter and aid becoming more permanent and adding to the problem was great. And donors had to be conscious that the media and donor attention to one crisis lasts only so long; attention will turn, all too soon, to the next disaster on our TV screens.

Finally, the reports stressed the vital importance of being prepared for crises such as the 2004 tsunami, and to have arrangements in place both for prevention and for more rapid response. Ireland took these recommendations seriously and by the time the Government published its 2006 White Paper on Irish Aid the lines of its approach to disasters were spelled out.[5]

The White Paper pledged that Ireland would provide "flexible and timely funding to local, Irish and international organisations that demonstrate a clear capacity to provide effective humanitarian assistance in a manner that is responsive to local needs and adheres to humanitarian principles." Addressing the coordination issue, it stated that "we will support the unique coordinating role of the UN and, when possible, the Government of the affected country." The White Paper also pledged support for developing countries in implementing measures to reduce the risk and minimize the human cost of humanitarian disasters, and for initiatives aimed at improving the capacity of developing countries, Irish and international NGOs, and international and multilateral organizations to prepare for and respond to humanitarian crises. It committed Ireland to linking disaster mitigation and long-term development.

As a way of putting these principles into practice, a Rapid Response Initiative was launched. It called for:

- the pre-positioning and transport of humanitarian supplies to disaster areas;

- the creation of a roster of highly skilled individuals, from the public and private sectors, including from the Defence Forces for deployment at short notice to emergency situations;

- enhancing the emergency capacities of international humanitarian response agencies and mechanisms.

In the years that followed, all of these initiatives were put in place. Stocks of nonfood items have been pre-positioned; the roster of skilled personnel has been created; and personnel have been frequently deployed to disaster areas. Ireland has acknowledged the key coordinating role of the Office for the Coordination of Humanitarian Affairs (OCHA) and contributed substantial funding to it and to the Central Emergency Relief Fund (CERF). (Ireland was a founder contributor to CERF; it has contributed $115 million since its creation in 2006 and remains the seventh-largest donor.) Irish Aid has formed strategic alliances with OCHA, WFP, and the International Committee of the Red Cross (ICRC). It has also streamlined its relations with those NGOs in Ireland that have the capacity to respond to disasters.

So, when the economic downturn happened in 2008 Ireland already had the policies and approaches in place to respond effectively. Of course, as indicated above, the size of the contributions to disaster relief had to be reduced—there was no alternative given Ireland's financial crisis. But the policies and strategies adopted in the mid-2000s have been implemented and even, in some cases, further developed.

A signal of Ireland's intentions was the publication by Irish Aid of a Humanitarian Relief Policy in 2009.[6] This document describes the context of work in disaster and sudden-onset emergency situations as fitting within Irish Aid's fundamental objective: poverty reduction. It sets out four basic principles that guide its humanitarian work:

1. **Humanity,** meaning the centrality of saving human lives and alleviating suffering wherever it is found.

2. **Impartiality,** meaning the provision of assistance solely on the basis of need, without discrimination between or within affected populations.

3. **Neutrality,** meaning that humanitarian assistance must not favor any side in an armed conflict or other dispute where such assistance is provided.

4. **Independence,** meaning the autonomy of humanitarian objectives from the personal, political, publicity, economic, military, or other objectives that any government or agency may hold with regard to areas where humanitarian assistance is being implemented.

The context for Ireland's approach to humanitarian assistance was the belief that combating hunger, in all its forms, is a top priority. Ireland has been to the forefront of the worldwide fight against hunger, having set up a Hunger Task Force in 2006. In 2010 Ireland joined with the U.S. Government to launch the "1,000 Days Initiative" focused on tackling undernutrition in the first thousand days of a child's life. And where does the specter of hunger raise itself so clearly as in a disaster situation?

★ ★ ★

Whether or not these policies and principles have been effective can be judged in the case of Ireland's response to three major challenges since the economic downturn: the Haiti earthquake, the Pakistan floods, and the famine in the Horn of Africa.

In January 2010 Haiti suffered a devastating earthquake. The death toll was similar to that in the 2004 tsunami—some 230,000 dead and 300,000 injured. The tragedy of the Haiti earthquake was particularly poignant as it was such a poverty-stricken country with hundreds of thousands of its people already living in abject conditions. Haiti was already facing huge development challenges with 80 percent of its people living below the poverty line and the worst income inequality indicators in the Western hemisphere.

Ireland did not have close ties to Haiti—its two largest NGOs, Concern and Trócaire, had modest programs there and, as ever, a few Irish missionaries were working in the country. And there were some Irish business links. But Haiti tugged at the heartstrings of the Irish people as previous disasters in other parts of the world had. Donations poured in to the NGOs and there was an expectation that the Government would play its part.

Two days after the earthquake, the Government authorized the dispatch of 83 tonnes of nonfood items from its pre-positioned stockpiles to Port-au-Prince. These included plastic sheeting, blankets, jerry cans, mosquito nets, and kitchen sets—some of the most urgently identified needs in the immediate aftermath of the earthquake.

The Government was also able to announce that CERF was one of the first mechanisms to respond to the crisis, thanks to the contributions made by Ireland and the other pooled donors. CERF allocated $10 million the morning after the earthquake and a further $15 million two days later.

A small technical team from Irish Aid went to Haiti in the fortnight after the disaster to establish where best Ireland could assist. The recommendations that the technical team made were in line with the policies described above: they recommended transferring further immediate relief from the pre-positioned stocks; stressed the need to have a speedy move from emergency relief to the recovery stage and to think in terms of a three-year time frame for this; the importance of channeling assistance through a limited number of partners with a proven track record and demonstrated capacity to help; active engagement with Haiti's national and local capacity; full participation in established coordination structures.

The technical team also concluded that as its assistance moved to the next phase Irish Aid should avoid diluting its contribution and should focus instead on a limited number of sectors: water, sanitation, and hygiene; shelter; and early recovery and protection.

As far as coordination was concerned, the team came away with mixed impressions; the clusters approach worked in some, but not all, areas while top-level leadership was only partially successful (a big blow was the fact that many of the UN personnel in Haiti themselves fell victim during the quake).

When the Haiti Donor Conference met in New York in March 2010, Ireland pledged $13 million. By 2012 it was able to report that it had expended 90 percent of that funding, mainly on the provision of clean water, sanitation, shelter, and housing through UNICEF and through the Irish NGOs Concern, GOAL, Plan, World Vision, and Haven. (Ireland, it might be mentioned, is proud of the fact that it honors the pledges it makes at such donor conferences. Some of the donors make grand pledges but do not deliver: of the $4.5 billion pledged at the conference only $2.8 billion has actually been disbursed.)

People I spoke to in Irish Aid felt that their response to the Haiti earthquake validated the policies that were adopted on disaster response. The ability to draw down supplies from the pre-positioned stocks, the rapid action of CERF to bring significant funding to bear, deployments from the Rapid Response Corps, the report from Irish Aid's own technical team, the focus on the niche areas of shelter, water, and sanitation—all were felt to have made a genuine impact on addressing a terrible disaster.

The close relationship between Irish Aid and the NGOs was also a very positive factor. Two innovative schemes that Irish Aid put in place have proved successful and have cemented the relationship in the area of disaster response. First, the Emergency Response Fund provides startup funding for five Irish NGOs (Concern, Trócaire, GOAL, Plan, World Vision) for use in the event of a sudden-onset emergency. The amount involved, while modest, enables these organizations to act quickly if a disaster occurs early in the year. The scheme, established by Irish Aid as part of its GHD commitments to have pre-positioned funds in place so as to enable timely response by its partner agencies, proved its value in the case of Haiti.

Second, the Humanitarian Policy Plans scheme allows the larger NGOs with a proven track record to sit down with Irish Aid and discuss their priorities for the year ahead. Some disasters, such as Haiti, are sudden-onset but many emergencies are more chronic in that they are the result of protracted crises arising from conflict or repeated droughts or flooding compounded by climate change, or a combination of the two. Under the Humanitarian Policy Plans scheme, the NGOs can get an indicative allocation of funding subject to the submission of specific proposals. This gives them an idea of the order of funding they will receive. Irish Aid benefits in that it gets a better sense of the particular strengths of different NGOs, their areas of expertise, regional knowledge, and so on.

Disaster of a different kind struck Pakistan in August 2010: extensive flooding across the country triggered an unprecedented humanitarian emergency. Some 20 million people were affected and the death toll reached 2,000. As in the case of Haiti, historical links between

Ireland and Pakistan have not been deep but, in this case also, the Irish people responded with generous private contributions.

Ireland was one of the first countries to respond. In the early days of the disaster, the minister of state in charge of Irish Aid convened an emergency meeting of Irish humanitarian NGOs and announced that Ireland would provide funding through OCHA, WFP, and UNICEF, as well as through Irish NGOs.

Two airlifts of pre-positioned emergency supplies were made to Pakistan, the second of which was the single-largest humanitarian airlift ever undertaken by Ireland. Shelter, water, and sanitation equipment were provided for 33,000 people. Ireland's support for CERF was again borne out in that CERF allocated $40 million to disaster response in Pakistan.

One unusual intervention came when the BBC World Service in Pakistan ran out of funds for a much-needed provision of information by radio and turned to Irish Aid for help. A donation of €50,000 helped to keep the program going and ensured that the affected populations continued to receive important information in Urdu and Pashto on ways in which they could receive help or cope with a very difficult situation.

Haiti and Pakistan posed unusual challenges for Irish Aid in that they occurred in the context of complex political situations, in countries with which Ireland had few links. In the case of Haiti, a major obstacle was the already very weak systems and poor governance; in Pakistan security was a continuing problem.

A more typical place for Irish involvement was the Horn of Africa, a region that Ireland has been assisting for several decades. In 2011 an already serious food security situation there came to a head. The failure of seasonal rains and successive droughts led to one of the most severe food crises in sixty years. Over 13 million people in drought-stricken areas of Djibouti, Ethiopia, Kenya, and Somalia were affected. The epicenter of the crisis was in southern Somalia where famine conditions brought back memories of the 1992 famine.

President Mary Robinson's visit to Somalia in 1992, the first by a western Head of State, is an iconic moment for Ireland's involvement with humanitarian assistance. Ireland took the lead then in bringing the catastrophe to world attention and made a substantial contribution through humanitarian aid, engagement by NGOs and volunteers, and Defence Force participation in the UN peacekeeping operations.

In the summer of 2011 images of starving children once again filled the TV screens. Robinson visited Somalia again, this time as International President of Oxfam, together with the heads of Concern and Trócaire. That visit served to spark greater interest in a public that had largely grown weary of the endless conflict in Somalia, a country that comes as close to the definition of a failed state as could be imagined.

It is worth making the point that the symbolism of a visit by an internationally respected figure like Robinson is an important contribution that a small country like Ireland can make. Both of her visits—some twenty years apart—helped to galvanize international interest in the plight of Somalia.

In order to ensure regional coverage and an appropriate overall response, Irish Aid sent out two technical teams to the Dadaab refugee camp in Kenya and the Dollo Ado camp in Ethiopia in July and August 2011 to see how best Ireland could help. Complicating the environmental aspect was the security/conflict situation in Somalia with the Al-Shabaab militants banning Western aid agencies from delivering supplies. The devastating combination of war and drought led to huge numbers of Somalis fleeing across the border. UNHCR estimated that 1.8 million people—almost a quarter of Somalia's population—were uprooted as a result.

Media focus concentrated on the Somali refugees who fled across the border into Kenya, and in particular to the Dadaab camp there. But the drought wrought havoc in Ethiopia and Kenya also. The technical teams made a series of recommendations that shaped Irish Aid's response. Two major airlifts of emergency water and shelter materials were carried out to help Concern and UNHCR with their activities in Somalia and the Dadaab refugee camp. Nineteen members of the Rapid Response Corps were deployed to assist humanitarian agencies.

So far, Ireland has allocated almost €16 million to the Horn of Africa relief effort, making Ireland, in per capita terms, a significant donor to the region. The total is likely to rise to €20 million in 2012 following a pledge at the summit on the Horn of Africa in New York in September 2011.

As well as concentrating on water and shelter, the team found that protection was a major issue, with the rates of rape and gender-based violence in the Dadaab camp and elsewhere very high. Women and girls were vulnerable in their flight and in the camps when they went to collect firewood or food. As a result, Ireland has advocated the appointment of suitably trained and experienced personnel within the Kenyan police to deal with the problem and has urged all stakeholders to put in place appropriate awareness, prevention, detection, and investigative strategies. Ireland has funded the provision of medical and psychological support for victims.[7]

Crucially, Ireland had also been ahead of the curve in terms of its overall funding response, having already been involved in supporting longer-term preventive work across the region. Irish Aid has invested in Ethiopia's Productive Safety Nets Programme and in the Humanitarian Programme Plans and the UN-managed Common Humanitarian Fund in Somalia. Important lessons are being drawn from this experience in shaping Ireland's response to this year's food crisis in the Sahel, notably the need to strengthen vulnerable people's coping mechanisms to withstand climate and other shocks.

Conclusions

To sum up: the quality of Ireland's disaster response has remained high even if the amount of funding available has fallen due to the economic downturn. I used to be skeptical at meetings of donors (the EU Directors-General meetings in Brussels for example, or the DAC meetings in Paris) when I would hear donors arguing that it was the quality of their aid delivery that counted. My suspicions would be aroused since that kind of language was sometimes used to distract attention away from a country's failure to reach volume targets. It was often a case of making a virtue out of necessity. It is true that the volume of Ireland's aid has fallen. But I believe that the emphasis on quality reflects a genuine wish to continue to search for ways to do disaster and emergency response better.

Professor Helen O'Neill, one of Ireland's most experienced commentators on development issues, publishes an annual report on the Irish Aid program. In her review of the performance in 2010 she paid particular attention to emergency response. She concluded:

> Irish Aid has been developing an increasingly integrated and coherent approach to providing assistance in emergency and recovery situations. It is no longer merely reactive to requests from NGOs and international agencies for funding. It has developed its own policy for strategic engagement with these partners and networks. Coherence now characterises the work of Irish Aid in its emergency and recovery work on both the bilateral and multilateral sides of the programme.[8]

What are the reasons that Ireland continues to deliver a quality product? The factors that combine to make this possible are worth identifying, as all donor countries share the wish to respond effectively and give value for their tax dollar. If I were to sum up the chief reasons why Ireland continues to have a good record on disaster response I would single out:

Having a well-thought-out humanitarian response policy. Most people's reflex to emergencies is to want to help, and to go into action quickly. But experience has shown that the risk of ineffective—even inappropriate—response to disasters is high. The time and nature of disasters may be unpredictable but they will certainly happen and having a clearly thought-out humanitarian response plan in place is essential.

Interest in, and commitment to, best practice. Ireland is a strong supporter of and contributor to the OECD DAC and is a member of best practice groups such as the GHD, the Like Minded Group and the Nordics+. As an EU member Ireland plays a part in the deliberations in Brussels on the EU's development policies. Discussion in these fora leads to sharing of experience—and learning from mistakes. Most of all, it enables a donor to stay abreast of best practice.

Being prepared. Pre-positioning of supplies is a key factor that enables Ireland to respond quickly. So too has been support for CERF.

Strong partners. Irish Aid works closely with a small group of leading organizations that have a proven track record: ICRC and the Red Crescent, WFP, and UNHCR. These organizations will always be better placed to make major interventions than smaller donors and they have a highly professional approach. Ireland has formed strategic alliances with all three and has kept track of their activities through regular consultations and, in the case of WFP and UNHCR, membership of their governing boards.

The other vital partners of Irish Aid in emergencies are the country's NGOs. Ireland is blessed with a strong NGO sector that has responded over several decades to major disasters and which can be relied on to deliver effect assistance. The three largest—Concern, Trócaire, and GOAL—are regarded as serious players internationally, and there are lots of others.

Coordination. The need for effective coordination in emergencies has long been apparent. Ireland's decision, as spelled out in the 2006 White Paper, to look to the UN as the chief coordinating body has been an important plank of the country's approach to emergencies. OCHA is recognized as the key player.

Niche areas. These are key for small donors where there is demonstrated need and where they have something to offer. In the three emergencies described above, Irish Aid was able to offer support to shelter and sanitation (Haiti), to education (Pakistan, especially in the postemergency phase), and to protection (Horn of Africa). As well as meeting clear needs, the focus in these cases played to Ireland's strengths. Protection is an example: Ireland has a good record in the fight against gender-based violence. A unique grouping of state bodies involved in development work, including the armed forces who participate in UN and other peacekeeping missions, NGOs, and human rights organizations came together in 2004 to form the Irish Gender Based Violence Consortium.

Prevention. Ireland's main contribution to the vital and still rather neglected aspect of disaster prevention is made through strengthening its partner countries' resilience. The aim of long-term development is to make countries and peoples more resilient and less vulnerable to extreme weather events. Improving governance is intended to lessen the risk of conflict. Emergencies do not arise from drought or conflict alone: much of Irish Aid's development work in its program countries is aimed specifically at building up communities' resilience to shocks in advance of their taking place.

Strong public support. Probably the most important single requirement for assistance to continue in times of a donor's economic difficulty is to maintain public support. It would be understandable in such a situation that the public's concerns should turn to home, especially when the debate about the Government's annual budget kicks in. The struggle to get a sufficient aid budget for Ireland to play its part will continue as the austerity measures needed to tackle Ireland's economic ills will continue. So far, public support for giving money to those far less well off than the people of Ireland remains steady. It helps that there is agreement across the political spectrum that Ireland should continue to play its part. One way of keeping support strong is to demonstrate that what the donor is doing represents value for money. Even before the economic downturn I noticed a greater demand on the Irish public's part for value for money in the aid program. There is far more scrutiny these days—rightly—and far more public awareness. Irish people, as in the rest of the world, know more today about disasters, even in the remotest parts of the world, thanks to the internet and the social media. The public's interest in their Government responding in a humane way that is effective is as great as ever. But there is no tolerance for unfocused aid interventions, however well-intentioned. Grandstanding won't wash.

Disaster response is a complex, multifaceted issue. It is a discipline within, but also distinct from, the broader field of development aid. It calls for special skills and mind-sets that are different from those required for long-term development. And, like all areas of development, the strategies required to deliver it well are evolving as better and more efficient ways are found.

Ireland has had to live with the challenge of delivering a good program of disaster response with smaller funding than before the economic downturn. That situation is unlikely to change in the short term; the heady days of the Celtic Tiger when Ireland could rank sixth among donors are gone. But the scorecard to date reads well. Here is the OECD's 2011 midterm review again:

> Ireland ensures a coordinated approach to disaster risk reduction and flexible responses to recovery and transition environments. Ireland has played a more prominent role in international fora since the last peer review (2009), co-chairing the Good Humanitarian Donorship initiative in 2009–10, and its advocacy has focused on the safety and security of humanitarian workers, information sharing at European level . . . and the governance of multilateral agencies. The aims of its advocacy are the advancement of good practice, strengthening of the global humanitarian system; professionalization of the GHD principles, active multilateralism, and increased learning opportunities.

The impulse to help the poorest runs deep in the Irish psyche. It has its roots in a historical sense of what it is to be on the receiving end and in the belief in helping your neighbor. That is not something that is likely to fade anytime soon.[9]

What Can Modern Society Learn from Indigenous Resiliency?

MARGARETA WAHLSTROM

The latest Global Platform on Disaster Risk Reduction in 2011 found that "a lot of knowledge about climate adaptation is not reaching those who need it the most"—how much more of a challenge is it then to get information, good practices, and capacity-building tools into the hands of indigenous communities using nonmainstream languages, so that they can adapt what's been learned to their ways of life? This challenge is alluded to in the international blueprint for disaster risk reduction agreed and endorsed by all United Nations Member States, the Hyogo Framework for Action (HFA) which prioritizes the use of knowledge, innovation, and education to build a culture of safety and resilience at all levels. The HFA Hyogo Framework Priority No. 3 recommends "Provid[ing] easily understandable information on disaster risk and protection options, especially to citizens in high-risk areas, to encourage and enable people to take actions to reduce risk and build resilience. The information should incorporate relevant traditional and indigenous cultural heritage and be tailored to different target audiences, taking into account cultural and social factors."

It is well recognized among policymakers and academics that indigenous peoples are more vulnerable than most to the factors driving risk such as poverty, bad planning, poor governance, prejudice, environmental degradation, and forced migration to cities and towns. Indigenous people also have something to teach modern communities about resilience and practices that protect environment and the community. However, many indigenous communities, pushed to the limits of their traditional lifestyles, have changed and may also adopt harmful practices that impact negatively on ecosystems for their survival.

Another important reality check is "scaling up." In a continuous search for viable alternatives to the consumer patterns that deplete natural resources and increase vulnerability, traditional practices offer inspiration to explore methods, but on a scale that is limited in space and habitat. The challenge is to find out how and what can be scaled to apply to today's urban communities that are different socially and economically from the indigenous communities.

Indigenous communities in many ways define resilience. How else would you describe a community that has preserved its institutions and ways of life over centuries other than as resilient? Yet, in other aspects, indigenous peoples, numbering some 370 million in ninety countries, are among the most vulnerable to natural and man-made hazards.

Some of the most disaster-prone countries in the world are also countries in which the indigenous people are a significant percentage of the overall population. The Instituto Indigenista Interamericano reckons that indigenous people constitutes 66 percent of the population in Guatemala, 63 percent in Bolivia, and 40 percent in Peru and Ecuador.

The range and intensity of hazards faced by indigenous communities is increasing with climate variability and more freak and extreme weather events. The Navajo Nation, for instance, is facing one of the longest droughts in recorded history, while at the other end of the extreme Pacific Islanders face the challenges of rising sea levels and increasingly intense typhoons.

As in all communities around the world, vulnerability to hazards among indigenous peoples is inextricably linked to socioeconomic development choices. The locations and structures that indigenous people live in may contribute to the risks. In too many indigenous communities development choices are not the community's choices. The forest fires that plague the peoples of Borneo—destroying crops and damaging health—can often be traced to large-scale land conversion. In other countries, forced relocation and dispossession has pushed people onto unfamiliar and inhospitable lands. And it is not a coincidence that indigenous lands are often selected as sites for toxic waste dumps.

Socioeconomic drivers of risk such as pervasive poverty, environmental degradation, and limited access to health care are pervasive in many indigenous communities.

Still it would be wrong to cast indigenous people as helpless victims because their endurance tells us that is not the case. Often theirs is the story of survival through adversity. So, how can this resilience be explained? Equipped with knowledge accumulated through generations of observation, many indigenous communities benefit from the hard-learned lessons of their ancestors. Some have resulted in resilient building designs that have withstood blowing winds and trembling earth.

The government of Bhutan, for example, has undertaken to examine their own construction practices and to learn from other cultures and share their insights internationally. In some cases, this entails blending the old with the new. In India, advice on bringing out the best of different knowledge systems and building disaster-resilient structures is available in the *Guidelines for Earthquake Resistant Non-Engineered Construction* report—such approaches exemplify the principal of doing more with less.[1]

In many indigenous communities, the accumulated knowledge stems from intimate observation of their environment. Native Hawaiians, for example, have long been able to identify dozens of types of winds and storms, even anticipating what we now recognize as the onset of the El Niño-Southern Oscillation. Local knowledge saved the lives of many villagers on the island of Simulue during the 2004 Indian Ocean tsunami. It is no surprise that when indigenous Dayak community leaders designed a training program for fire prevention in Borneo, they set "learning to observe local forest and temperature conditions" as the first learning objectives.

One of the distinguishing features of resilience is found in the ways that communities recover. Indigenous communities have strong adaptive capacities. Extensive and enduring social networks that bind communities provide the foundations of a social safety net. The ways that indigenous communities establish networks are translated into broader national and international settings. Grassroots and indigenous women first met in Antigua Guatemala, for example, in 2008 and shared their experiences in making their communities less vulnerable to disasters. They drafted a document outlining their plans for increased cooperation among themselves and for greater participation in the disaster risk reduction plans of their respective governments. This is a very practical example of how indigenous knowledge can be immediately transformed into learning for the wider society.

The history of indigenous peoples includes periods of resistance and cooperation with populations that have sought to dominate them. Article 3 of the United Nations Declaration on the Rights of Indigenous Peoples states, "Indigenous peoples have the right to self-determination. By virtue of that right they freely determine their political status and freely pursue their economic, social and cultural development." Indigenous peoples have long struggled for the right to say no to short-sighted development schemes and to promote their own approaches to development. Determination of balanced approaches to growth and development is not a right held exclusively by indigenous peoples.

The cultural diversity of the world's indigenous peoples is an asset to us all in our various efforts to build resilient communities and nations. Diverse ways of life, values, and knowledge systems can reduce our collective fragility and in fact enrich us. It is however important to base this on the understanding that the right of indigenous populations to participate in the economic and social progress of countries is a fundamental one—and a necessary starting point.

This section details the plight of several sectors of society that bear unusual burdens in any disaster. Women and children are always most vulnerable. Until recently, almost no attention was paid to a forgotten, and ignored, group who suffer from noncommunicable diseases. Their dependence on medications and medical care is disrupted and, without proper planning, they silently die in large numbers.

There are, however, new tools, including advanced technology and the use of modern media, which offer creative options that go beyond current practices in disaster relief. In addition to the human damage that follows disasters, part of our cultural soul, the essence of our civilization, can be damaged and lost. This critical dimension deserves attention in both preparedness and response. The final chapter in this section focuses on educating a cadre of men and women in the realities of fieldwork as experienced in disasters so that they are capable of delivering a coordinated and effective response.

Providing for the Most Vulnerable in the Twenty-First Century

FLAVIA BUSTREO, M.D.

Whether it was Iraq after the first Gulf war, Sarajevo during the
siege, or Sudan during the protracted conflict, it was always the
eyes of women and children that conveyed to me the horror and
tragedy of conflicts. It is through their eyes that I am writing this
chapter and for their health that I have committed twenty years
of my professional life.

When discussing disasters, humanitarian response, reconstruction,
and risk reduction, it is appropriate to begin with women's and children's health. Women and children usually are the most affected by
civil conflict, displacement, disaster, and war. As the Beijing Agenda
for Global Action on Gender-Sensitive Disaster Risk Reduction (2009)
set out: "We are fully aware that women comprise 70 percent of the
world's poor and women are more vulnerable to the impact of disaster
due to the existing socio-economic, political and cultural disadvantages."[1] Millions of children throughout the world are subject to crises
that last for years and that compromise their well-being and increase
their vulnerabilities.[2] Both women and children are also vulnerable to
violence and sexual abuse in crisis situations.

Women today also increasingly help to shape the world in public are-
nas. They play an important role in art, business, development, human
rights, politics, science, and technology. Women also shape the world in
private spaces, and continue to remain the primary carers of the family.
In disasters, women often continue in their roles as primary caregivers
for children, the elderly, and the injured. Women's ability to care for
themselves and their families is limited by the loss of livelihoods and

support, sometimes caused by the deaths or displacement of male heads of households. Children are looked to as the future of our world, and ensuring their health, education, and flourishing must be considered a fundamental human commitment.

And yet for many women and children today even survival, their basic right to life, is a challenge. Every day, almost 1,000 women[3] die while giving birth and around 21,000 children[4] under the age of five die from preventable and treatable causes. In disasters, these health and life vulnerabilities of women and children are multiplied. A World Health Organization (WHO) analysis reports on "adverse reproductive outcomes following disasters including early pregnancy loss, premature delivery, stillbirths, delivery-related complications and infertility."[5] For children in disasters, addressing malnutrition, the need for safe water and immunization, child protection from violence, and access to education and play are critical challenges.[6]

This chapter focuses on the two Millennium Development Goals (MDGs) that are related to the challenge of preventing and reducing maternal and child mortality. Addressing these two goals will help increase the resilience of women and children and of families and communities in times of disasters, and provide the necessary support for the reconstruction and development of affected societies.

Promising Commitments for Women's and Children's Health

After the child-survival revolution in the 1980s and early 1990s,[7] along with the Safe Motherhood Initiative in Nairobi in the 1980s,[8] the interest and commitment to maternal and child health in the humanitarian sphere began to decrease. But in the year 2000, the MDGs, which were agreed upon by all 191 United Nations (UN) Member States, included a central focus on poverty, development, and health, with an emphasis on women's and children's health.[9] Academics played a critical role in this renaissance. There were landmark articles that appeared in the *British Medical Journal* and the *Lancet*; the latter's focus on child survival, maternal mortality, and newborn survival brought the attention of policymakers and leaders to the fact that not enough progress was being made. The WHO also contributed to the renaissance in 2005 with their report entitled *Make Every Mother and Child Count*.[10]

In 2005, the WHO launched the Partnership for Maternal, Newborn and Child Health (PMNCH), which currently has more than 450 members.[11] It comprises a number of partners in different constituency groups: academics, governments, multilateral organizations, donors, professionals associations, nongovernmental organizations, and the private sector.

But the moment the renaissance really came together occurred in 2010. For the first time, the Group of Eight (G8)[12] launched a specific initiative on maternal and child health. The initiative was called "Muskoka," after the town in Canada where the meeting was held.[13] In the same year, at an African Union summit held in Kampala, Uganda, the African heads of state decided that there would be a report every year on the situation and progress of the health of women and children in Africa until 2015.[14]

Most importantly in 2010, the United Nations General Assembly, under the leadership of the Secretary-General Ban Ki-moon, launched the Global Strategy for Women's and Children's Health.[15] There were unprecedented commitments totalling $40 billion by constituency groups including governments, private sector organizations, academics, and developing organizations, with additional significant policy and service commitments to improve women's and children's health.

The Size of the Problem

MDG 4 aims to reduce child mortality and MDG 5 to improve maternal health and both are closely related to a number of other MDGs. They very much relate to MDG 3 (to promote gender equality and empower women) and also to MDG 2 (to achieve universal primary education). We know very well that educating young women can help with the health and survival of their children.

So what are the specific targets of MDGs 4 and 5? For MDG 4 the target is to reduce the under-five mortality rate by two-thirds between

1990 and 2015. MDG 5 has two targets: a) reduction of the maternal mortality rate by three-quarters between 1990 and 2015, and b) universal access to reproductive health (this was added in 2007 and was not part of the original target).

When looking at MDG 4 and the under-five mortality rate, there has been progress. In Figure 1 the light grey shows the countries that are on track, dark grey shows where there is insufficient progress, and black shows where there is little progress. The figure also shows countries that continue to experience some increases in child mortality due to HIV/AIDS or conflict situations (see Figure 1). It is a similar picture for the newborn mortality rate. This is important, as in the past the linkage between mothers and newborns and mothers and children had somehow been missed. Actors and partners were operating separately to address the health of children and somehow the newborn population was falling through the cracks, and the care that was given to newborns immediately after delivery was part of a different program. In fact, poor neonatal health accounts for more than 40 percent of child mortality for children under the age of five. There are preterm births, asphyxia, sepsis, pneumonia, congenital anomalies, diarrheal diseases,

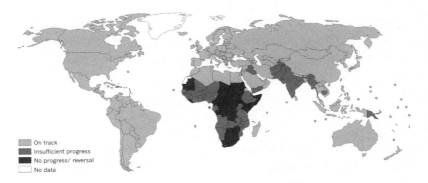

On track
Insufficient progress
No progress/ reversal
No data

Figure 1. MDG 4: Under-Five Mortality Rates; Little Progress in Africa, Insufficient Progress in Asia

Sources: UNICEF, WHO, World Bank, and UN DESA/Population Division, *Levels and Trends in Child Mortality* (New York: UNICEF, 2010); and White Ribbon Alliance, "White Ribbon Atlas of Birth" (November 2010 edition). Available from www.whiteribbonalliance.org.

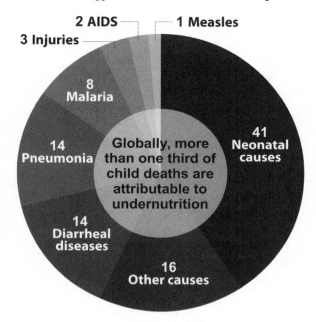

Figure 2. MDG 4: Main Causes of Death among Children under Five, 2008 (%)
Source: United Nations, *Millennium Development Goals Report 2010* (New York: United Nations, 2010). Available from www.un.org/en/mdg/summit2010/pdf/ MDG%20Report%202010%20En%20r15%20-low%20res%2020100615%20-.pdf.

tetanus, and other neonatal causes, of which HIV/AIDS is playing an increasing part due to the epidemic increase in the later part of the last century (see Figure 2).

For MDG 5(a), the target of maternal mortality rate, the picture is very similar, with the highest maternal mortality rate occurring in Sub-Saharan Africa. An analysis of the world's total maternal mortality rate indicates a decline at an annual rate of 2.3 percent. While this is a positive development, it is not nearly enough if we want to reach the target of 5.5 percent that is needed to reach MDG 5 (see Figure 3 and Table 1).

MDG 5(b), which relates to reproductive health, has as its indicator access to equal rights for family planning. The unmet need for contraception is higher in the countries where the maternal mortality rate is

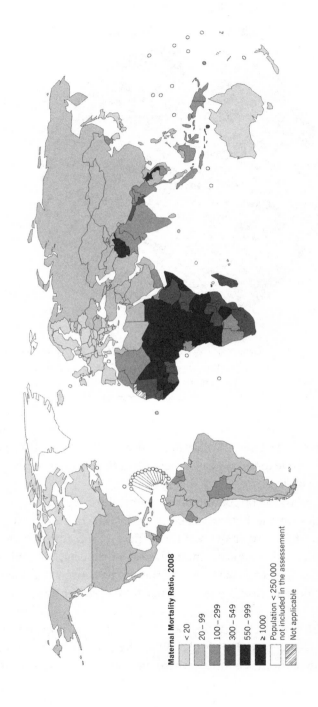

Maternal Mortality Ratio, 2008

- < 20
- 20 – 99
- 100 – 299
- 300 – 549
- 550 – 999
- ≥ 1000
- Population < 250 000 not included in the assessement
- Not applicable

Figure 3. MDG 5b: Maternal Mortality Ratio Is Still High

Source: WHO, UNICEF, UNFPA, and the World Bank, *Estimates of Maternal Mortality Levels and Trends 1990–2008* (Geneva: WHO, 2010).

Table 1. Global Maternal Mortality in 2008 with Average Annual Decline from 1990 to 2008

	MMR (2008) (UNCERTAINTY INTERVAL)	MATERNAL DEATHS (N) (2008)	AVERAGE ANNUAL DECLINE (%)
World (total)	260 (200, 370)	358,000	2.3 (2.1, 2.4)
Developed regions	14 (13, 16)	1700	0.8 (0.6, 1.0)
Countries of the CIS	40 (34, 48)	1500	3.0 (2.8, 3.1)
Developing regions	290 (220, 410)	355,000	2.3 (2.2, 2.5)
North Africa	92 (60, 140)	3400	5.0 (4.8, 5.1)
Sub-Saharan Africa	640 (470, 930)	204,000	1.7 (1.4, 1.9)
Asia	190 (130, 270)	139,000	4.0 (3.9, 4.1)
Latin America and the Caribbean	85 (72, 100)	9200	2.9 (2.6, 3.3)
Oceania	230 (100, 500)	550	1.4 (1.2, 1.3)
MDG target			5.5

Note: Numbers are rounded.

high (see Figure 4). For example, in Chad only 1.6 percent of married women use a modern form of contraception. The cause of maternal deaths worldwide include obstructed labor, abortion, and sepsis, all of which widely contribute to child mortality, while other causes, like HIV/AIDS, have a very disparate effect in different parts of the world.

This data summarizes the acceleration period to reach these 2015 targets. I am quite optimistic that acceleration can be achieved, but it must be noted that the countries that are not making progress are often those in conflict or postconflict situations, such as the Democratic Republic of Congo and Afghanistan.

A Continuum of Care for Mothers, Newborns, and Children

Conflicts increase women's and children's health-care needs, while at the same time reducing the health system's capacity to respond. All functions of the health system are affected by conflict. The disruption of the health system and other vital infrastructure prevents countries from ensuring the continuum of care for mothers, newborn, and children.

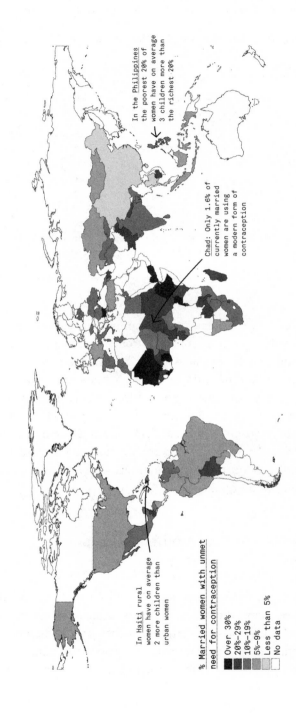

In the Philippines the poorest 20% of women have on average 3 children more than the richest 20%

Chad: Only 1.6% of currently married women are using a modern form of contraception

In Haiti rural women have on average 2 more children than urban women

% Married women with unmet need for contraception

- Over 30%
- 20%–29%
- 10%–19%
- 5%–9%
- Less than 5%
- No data

Figure 4. MDG 5b: The Unequal World of Family Planning

Source: White Ribbon Alliance, "White Ribbon Atlas of Birth" (November 2010 edition). Available from www.whiteribbonalliance.org.

This means quality services and care for women and children that start before pregnancy and extend through birth and postdelivery for both mother and baby are crucial. It is vital that these services continue after childbirth, through adolescence and into adulthood, through the provision of counselling and family planning. This continuum of care should be multifaceted, spanning across all stages of pregnancy and ranging from care in the home to care in the hospital (if necessary), with services for both the mother and child.

Observing these interventions along the continuum of care, we see that some of them have reached quite significant coverage (see Figure 5). For example, immunization interventions that can be delivered through campaigns or through a mass delivery of vitamin A have reached the significant level of 80 percent in the sixty-eight countries that account for 95 percent of maternal deaths (see Figure 5). However, other interventions, for example treating malaria in pregnant women, along with other well-known and established treatments of pneumonia and diarrhea of children under five, still remain under 50 percent (see Figure 5).

One other aspect that is very critical is equity. There needs to be a focus on equity because the poorest and most vulnerable women and children are the most difficult to reach. The overall coverage of these interventions can mask very high inequities. For example, a comparison of Zambia and Guatemala that examines the implementation of eight health interventions on average for women and children is misleading. Among the poorest women in Zambia, 55 percent are receiving these eight interventions; in Guatemala less than 40 percent of the poorest women are receiving these interventions whereas but the country's richest women receive 85 percent of these same interventions.

In other words, our analysis has to look across the interventions, but also across the different socioeconomic groups. Availability and social exclusion is one dimension—one of many—but it is a critical one. And looking at the different interventions we also found marked differences in the role this inequity played in the population, with respect to the poorest and the richest. For example, the gap between the richest and the poorest may be readily seen by measuring the number of pre- and postnatal visits, and the frequency of skilled attendants at

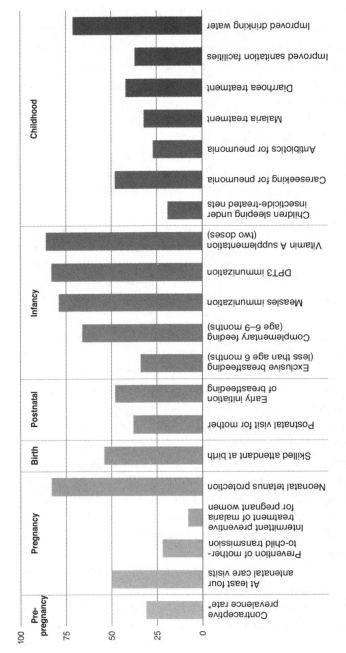

Figure 5. Coverage of Interventions along the Continuum of Care with Median National Coverage of Interventions across the Continuum of Care for 20 Countdown Interventions and Approaches in Countdown Countries, Most Recent Year since 2000 (%)

Target coverage value is not 100%.

Source: Countdown to 2015, *Countdown to 2015 Decade Report (2000–2010): Taking Stock of Maternal, Newborn, and Child Survival* (Geneva: Countdown to 2015, 2010). Available from www.countdown2015mnch.org/reports-and-articles/2010-decade-report.

delivery. With other interventions, however, such as Oral Rehydration Treatment (ORT) for diarrhea, the difference in access to treatment between the richest and the poorest was less marked.

We Lack Human Resources for Women's and Children's Health

One other aspect to note is how critical the work health force is in making progress for women's and children's health, especially in countries in conflict or postconflict situations. Data from the WHO Health Report in 2006 show a critical shortage of health-service providers, doctors, nurses, and especially midwives in the countries coloured in dark grey (see Figure 6). This shortage occurs in the same countries where there is the highest maternal mortality rate and where civil conflict strikes.

These statistics are hardly surprising, as human capital is typically the first to be affected by conflict. Health staff are lost due to insecu-

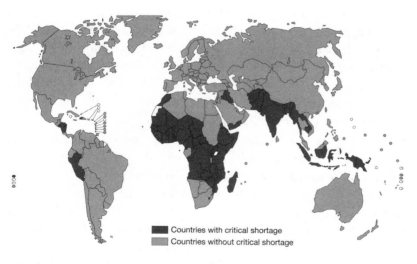

Countries with critical shortage
Countries without critical shortage

Figure 6. The Health Workforce: There Is a Critical Shortage of Doctors, Nurses, and Midwives in Fifty-Seven Countries
Source: WHO, *The World Health Report 2006: Working together for Health* (Geneva: WHO, 2006). Available from www.who.int/whr/2006/whro6_en.pdf.

rity, and there is a brain drain of doctors, particularly specialized physicians. One half of doctors and 80 percent of pharmacists left Uganda between 1972 and 1985.[16] In Mozambique, only 16 percent of doctors stayed after 1975.[17] In East Timor, the postreferendum violence severely affected the availability of health staff.[18] Even when local health staff remains, they face an increased workload due to conflict and often lack adequate supplies and equipment.[19]

Human resource challenges, therefore, remain a hurdle for many countries not yet "on track" to reach the MDGs. Solutions are being found in expanding the the number of skilled staff, improving skills and providing workers with new technologies, deploying staff to underserved communities, improving motivation, and shifting tasks to increase the capacity of available staff to provide needed services. Of the countries with available data, fifty-seven do not have the minimum level of staff recommended to provide the services required to reach coverage and mortality reduction targets.[20] Sub-Saharan Africa accounts for 50 percent[21] of the world's maternal and child deaths, but only 3 percent[22] of the world's health workers. India and Ethiopia have created new cadres of community workers to provide preventative and some curative services. Mozambique has used task shifting—successfully training and deploying clinical technicians to perform surgeries, including cesarean sections in the absence of sufficient obstetricians or surgeons, resulting in the survival of many at-risk mothers and babies.

There is a clear linkage between the density of health workers and maternal and infant mortality. Thailand is considered a success story in this area, and an excellent example of the progress they have made in reducing maternal mortality since 1940.[23] It certainly wasn't coincidental that when they scaled up midwifery training and when they focused on strengthening this resource, there was a reduction on maternal mortality rates.[24] The clinical role that health-care providers and mass-scale delivery provides has been improving, especially among maternal health, and demonstrates the linkage that exists between maternal mortality and the strength of the health system. In fact, it has been gradually accepted that maternal mortality is the litmus test to see whether health systems are actually strong.

More Money for Health and More Health for Money

The very distinguished Indian professor Vulimiri Ramalingaswami coined the famous phrase "more money for health and more health for money." This can be readily applied to maternal and child health.

Are we seeing more money for maternal and child health? Figure 7 shows government expenditures on health around the world; the countries in red spend less than $15 per person for health. There is clearly overlap between countries that are striving to make progress on maternal and child mortality reduction and the level of investment in health.

On the more positive side, there is data to support that even the poorest countries, like Malawi and Ethiopia, are increasing the level of domestic resources allocated to maternal and child health. For example, as Figure 8 shows, in Ethiopia the size of the light grey bar is getting smaller. This means that the proportion of reproductive and child health expenditures is increasingly financed by domestic resources and less by the external official development assistance (ODA) resources.

However, conflict affects both domestic and ODA resources allocated to health as funds are diverted to military and security activities. Chad, for example, one of the poorest countries in the world with very low social spending, was torn by persistent conflicts during 1965–87. During 1972–78, defense spending increased by 28 percent, while health spending increased only by 4 percent. During 1981–82, members of the Organization of African Unity raised about $237 million for a peacekeeping mission in Chad, more than the country's total allocation to health over a ten-year period.[25]

The flipside of the Ramalingaswami quote is "more health for the money," so part of our next challenge is to examine how the investments and commitments we have seen provide more resources to target countries with the highest needs and to produce better results. We can maximize impact through integration and link efforts to improve women's and children's health with efforts that are intended to tackle poverty, nutrition, and access to education. Education is critical, especially with regard to the effect that maternal education has on child mortality and sanitation (e.g., in the prevention of diarrheal diseases).

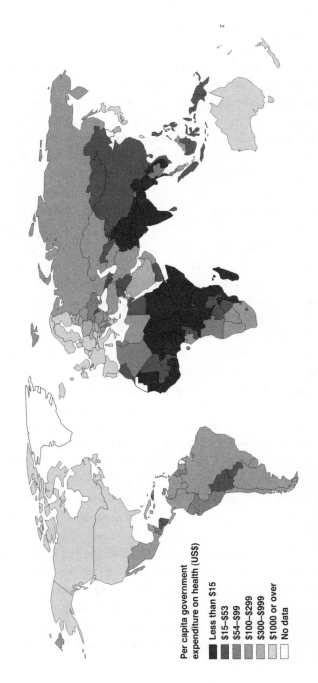

Figure 7. Governments' Expenditure on Health

Per capita government
expenditure on health (US$)

- Less than $15
- $15–$53
- $54–$99
- $100–$299
- $300–$999
- $1000 or over
- No data

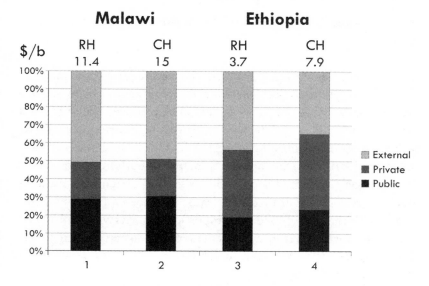

Figure 8. National Financial Flows Are More Important than ODA Even in the Poorest Countries

Source: Reproductive Health and Child Health Sub-Accounts ca 2005.

We can also maximize impact and achieve more health for the money through using innovation to increase efficiency and impact. There is a range of innovative approaches in leadership, results-based financing and public/private partnerships. Information technology can help us better communicate to frontline providers in real time about the needs of particular communities and can help better assess the rate of and reasons for maternal mortality, as well as measure birth rates across communities. Many countries are hampered by an inability to reliably gather and measure vital statistics. We can also maximize impact through making funding channels more efficient. One of the greatest examples of progress we have seen is the Paris Agreement, also known as the Paris Principles, where countries have agreed to a set of principles to provide assistance in making their funding more long-term, predictable, and harmonized.[26] Some instruments like the Global Alliance for Vaccines and Immunization, and the Global Fund are at the forefront of making these funding challenges more efficient.[27]

Progress Is Possible and There Are Examples of Success

Even in countries suffering protracted civil strife progress in maternal and child mortality is possible. For example, Sri Lanka, a low-income country, was for over twenty-five years in a protracted civil war which caused significant hardships for the population, environment, and the economy of the country. And yet Sri Lanka has successfully reduced maternal mortality. Starting with a maternal mortality ratio of 1,056 maternal deaths per 100,000 live births in 1947, by 1996 it was experiencing just twenty-four maternal deaths per 100,000 live births. During roughly the same period, the proportion of births with skilled birth attendants increased from 27 percent in 1940 to 89 percent in 1995. The following key actions helped to achieve this dramatic reduction in maternal mortality rates:

- A vast network of health infrastructure extending into rural areas was established by the 1950s to make health services more accessible. This included blood transfusion services. Services were also provided free of charge.

- Large cadres of professional midwives were trained and deployed both at the health facilities and in communities to attend to home deliveries. Additionally, midwives visited pregnant women at home and encouraged them to seek antenatal care and assistance during delivery.

- Family planning was integrated into maternal and child health services and offered as part of the basic package of services.

- A strong referral system ensured timely access to basic and comprehensive emergency obstetric and newborn services when necessary, backed by the availability of ambulances and telephones.

- Steps were taken to ensure that data needed to track progress was made available. Civil registration systems and health management information systems were established and strengthened. Maternal death reviews were instituted in the 1950s to identify the factors contributing to maternal deaths, enabling corrective actions. These reviews also allowed issues of quality of care to be addressed.

The Sri Lankan government's commitment led to a dramatic reduction in maternal mortality. Given that public expenditure on health care was low (on average less than 2 percent of GDP) during the 1950–99 period, this reduction cannot be attributed to a huge investment of funds. This indicates that other low-income countries with high maternal mortality, even during protracted civil strife, could also reduce maternal mortality with political commitment and the appropriate interventions.

The Challenges Ahead

In terms of the global effort to reach the MDGs related to maternal and child mortality, a significant focus must be placed on countries in conflict or postconflict situations. As we have seen, in those countries the mortality rates remain the highest, health systems are disrupted, health workers leave, and financial resources are diverted to the military. In terms of policy, one of the areas where we have been less successful in recent years is the multisectoral role of policies, for example, the International Labour Organization's Maternal Protection Convention, which is meant to protect women in the labor force by providing them with rights to maternity leave and job protection, as well as the right to return to work after maternity leave.[28] On the services-delivery side, one of the challenges ahead is how we progress from the vertical programs that are providing specific integration to integrated platforms that deliver services for women and children when and where they are needed, especially in a disaster situation.

Additionally, women's participation and empowerment are crucial. What we see is that when we put money in the hands of women, we achieve tremendous results. For example, when India's social protection scheme provided cash to women to provide them with both access to a health facility and the agency to decide to visit one, a tremendous increase in the number of women that were able and willing to go to a health facility during labor was seen. Finally, the funding transition— from dependency on ODA to sustainable domestic financing for those critical services—still presents a challenge, especially for the countries with the lowest incomes.

Conclusions

> Health is a fundamental human right. In countries where children
> die early and mothers die in the act of giving life, injustice breeds.
> —Dr. Julio Frenk, Dean, Harvard School of Public Health

The important goal we need to move toward is the highest attainable standards of health. The highest attainable standard of health for women and children, including in disaster, is a fundamental human right and should not depend on the geographical circumstances of where people are born. On this issue last year, we saw a very high engagement from the UN Human Rights Council when they passed a resolution on avoidable maternal death as an issue of human rights concern.

The linkage of health as a fundamental human right and the lack of that right leads to injustice. In countries where injustice breeds peace and stability cannot develop, and this is the vicious cycle we need to break. If we can save women from dying in childbirth and children from dying young, we create just societies that can grow and remain peaceful and prosperous.

Women and children are particularly vulnerable to the consequences of conflict and poverty. Not only does the effect of conflicts on women and child health constitute a violation of a fundamental human right, but it also presents serious impediments to creating and sustaining healthy, prosperous and stable societies. Unless the health needs of women and children in conflict-affected countries are addressed in an effective and stable manner, the prospects of achieving the MDGs of reducing maternal and child mortality will be limited.

Noncommunicable Diseases and the New Global Health

THOMAS J. BOLLYKY

When most people in developed countries think of the biggest health challenges confronting the developing world, they envision a small boy in a rural, dusty village beset by an exotic parasite or bacterial blight. But increasingly, that image is wrong. Instead, it is the working-age woman living in an urban slum in a middle-income country, suffering from diabetes, cervical cancer, or stroke—noncommunicable diseases (NCDs) that once confronted wealthy nations alone.

NCDs in developing countries are occurring more rapidly, arising in younger people, and leading to far worse health outcomes than ever seen in developed countries. This epidemic results from persistent poverty, unprecedented urbanization, and freer trade in emerging market nations, which have not yet established the health and regulatory systems needed to treat and prevent NCDs. According to the 2009 *Global Risks* report published by the World Economic Forum (WEF), these diseases pose a greater threat to global economic development than fiscal crises, natural disasters, transnational crime and corruption, or infectious disease.[1]

The international community has done little to help. Most donors remain focused on the battle against infectious diseases, reluctant to divert their funds. A recent United Nations General Assembly (UNGA) meeting devoted to NCDs produced few concrete measures. With the global economy still in decline and funding scarce, the chances of new effective cooperation seem smaller than ever.

Collective action on NCDs need not wait for UN endorsement, economic recovery, or a reallocation of money away from campaigns against infectious diseases. International diplomacy and the mobilization of massive amounts of development aid matter less in the fight against the NCD epidemic in developing countries than in HIV/AIDS and other recent global health efforts. Technical agencies, regional coordination, and adaptation of existing technologies and delivery platforms will matter more. The international community can make progress now by addressing those NCDs that are especially prevalent among poor people in developing countries and the particular needs of their governments to address these diseases. In doing so, it can help curtail avoidable sickness and death and set the precedent for action on other emerging global health challenges that share the same origins and devastating consequences for the world's poor as the NCD crisis.

Collectively Stalled

In 1996, a landmark World Health Organization (WHO) report on the global burden of disease concluded that NCDs would soon dwarf the burden of infectious diseases and maternal, perinatal, and nutritional conditions in low- and middle-income countries.[2] It was, at that time, a groundbreaking insight that contradicted long-standing views of NCDs as diseases of affluence, and the WHO report cautioned that the rapidity of this epidemiological transition and the very large numbers involved would pose serious challenges to health-care systems and the allocation of scarce resources.

After its 1996 report, WHO attempted to address the emerging global NCD crisis. Among other measures, WHO produced a Global Strategy for Prevention and Control of Noncommunicable Diseases (1999); established a WHO department dedicated to NCD control and prevention (2001); successfully negotiated the Framework Convention on Tobacco Control (2003); generated a Global Strategy on Diet, Physical Activity, and Health (2004); and released the 2008–2013 Action Plan for the Global Strategy for the Prevention and Control of Noncommunicable

Diseases (2008). Traction remained elusive, however, within a global health community otherwise occupied with HIV/AIDS, maternal and child health, and neglected diseases. As Rachel Nugent and Andrea Feigl have estimated, 70 percent of total donor funding for NCDs between 2004–8 came from just three sources, by far the largest of which was WHO itself. In 2007, donor funding for NCDs was less than 3 percent ($503 million out of $22 billion) of total global health donor funds.[3]

To address the persistent international community neglect of NCDs, Caribbean countries and a group of nongovernmental organizations (NGOs) led a successful effort to hold a UNGA high-level meeting on NCDs in September 2011. Organizers agreed that the meeting would address the challenges of NCDs worldwide but focus on cancer, diabetes, cardiovascular disease, and respiratory illnesses, in part because those diseases share four major risk factors: tobacco use, alcohol use, physical inactivity, and an unhealthy diet. The WHO produced a set of strategies to reduce these factors, estimating that it would cost approximately $11.4 billion per year to fund them in developing countries.[4] Expectations for the meeting were high. The only other UNGA high-level meetings on health have been on HIV/AIDS, which helped create the Global Fund to Fight AIDS, Tuberculosis, and Malaria and motivate donors to spend billions of dollars to put patients in the developing world on lifesaving drugs.

Hopes that the outcomes of the UN NCD high-level meeting would match those of its HIV/AIDS predecessors soon faded however. Infighting persisted among the NCD community over the exclusion of major disease groups, mental illnesses in particular. The donors that have dominated recent international responses to infectious diseases, such as the Bill and Melinda Gates Foundation, argued that the meeting could distract from existing global health initiatives and divert their funding.[5] With the tobacco, food and beverage, pharmaceutical, agriculture, and other industries potentially implicated, lobbying in advance of the meeting was intense.[6] Advance negotiations among UN Member States became bogged down in disagreements over whether to agree to NCD reduction targets and mandatory measures to contain these diseases worldwide. More than 130 countries, thirty heads of state, and hundreds of NGOs representing a bewildering array of diseases attended the high-level meeting. The streets outside the UN, however, remained empty of the masses of supporters that characterized the HIV/AIDS UN high-level meetings. With its focus on the worldwide rise in unhealthy lifestyles and inactivity, one public health colleague referred to the UN meeting as "the global couch potato conference."

The commitments that emerged from the UN high-level meeting were largely rhetorical. The resulting political declaration recognizes the "epidemic proportions" of NCDs and notes that countries can prevent them with cost-efficient public health measures, but does not mandate specific approaches or their adoption.[7] It endorses private-sector partnerships and the sharing of technical assistance between developed and developing countries, but designates no entity to undertake or fund this effort. The most concrete action mandated by the declaration is to shift the responsibility back to WHO, charging it with generating the voluntary disease and risk reduction targets upon which UN members could not agree, and asking UN members to "consider" these targets in developing their national NCD plans. The UNGA approval of the declaration was unanimous. A subsequent resolution of the WHO Executive Board revealed that WHO has been unable to achieve agreement among its 194 Member States on voluntary disease- and risk reduction targets and is likely to postpone the matter until the next World Health Assembly in May 2013.[8]

In the end, the high-level meeting helped mobilize the NGO community and broaden public recognition of the human and economic toll of NCDs worldwide, but produced, at least so far, limited resources and accountability for addressing that challenge. Several governments, of their own volition, introduced new regulations on trans fats and dietary salt.[9] Numerous corporations, such as PepsiCo, announced that they would launch voluntary initiatives to make their products healthier and donate funds to improve the treatment of NCDs.[10] Even so, frustrated supporters demanded a more comprehensive meeting to address the social and economic causes of NCDs worldwide.[11] Critics cited these modest results as proof that amid the global financial troubles and corporate lobbying, collective action on NCDs is impossible.[12]

The Original Sin of Taxonomy

The notion that a weak global economy and a conspiracy of industrial lobbyists prevented progress at the UN meeting is wrong. As currently pursued, international efforts on NCDs would also fail to generate support in a good economy—as they have since the WHO first reported the emerging epidemic of NCDs in 1996. The effectiveness of corporate lobbying at the UN meeting was a symptom of poorly conceived collective action on NCDs, not its cause.

The reasons for the lack of progress at the UN high-level meeting begin with the mislabeling of the diseases now known as NCDs. The classification originates with that 1996 landmark WHO global burden of disease report and was used to distinguish NCDs (Group II diseases) from communicable, maternal, perinatal, and nutritional conditions (Group I) and unintentional and intentional injuries (Group III). In addition to cancer, diabetes, cardiovascular diseases, and respiratory illnesses, NCDs include a wide array of conditions, such as skin diseases, congenital anomalies, mental disorders, rheumatoid arthritis, and dental decay.

Trying to address these diseases as a single class and on a global level has both broadened opposition and diffused support for effective action. On one hand, addressing NCDs as a single category has united a wide array of otherwise disconnected industries, from agriculture to pharmaceutical companies and restaurants, against global targets to reduce NCDs and their risk factors. On the other hand, it has made it difficult to mobilize governments and sufferers of NCDs worldwide around a specific and meaningful policy agenda. When NCDs are presented as imposing the same challenges in developed and developing countries alike, policymakers and potential donors are apt to conclude that they cannot be solved by international action and are simply the natural consequence of economic development.

The NCD designation is a misnomer for these diseases. As a class, NCDs are not all noncommunicable; some are spread by viruses, bacteria, and social practices. NCDs are also not, as some have claimed, diseases of affluence or gluttony, sloth, and intemperance; many are endemic. Nor are all NCDs chronic; some may be quickly cured with the appropriate health intervention. As a class, NCDs have little in common other than being the diseases that become more prevalent as a population reduces the plagues and parasites that kill children and adolescents. In short, NCDs are the diseases of those with longer lives. While this designation may lack the punch required for effective advocacy and fundraising, it gets at the heart of the forces driving the NCD crisis in developing countries today.

The Challenges of Living Longer

The reasons for the exploding NCD crisis in developing countries begin, paradoxically, with increased life expectancy. The greater availability of effective medical technologies, such as vaccines, and the improved diffusion of good public health practices, such as hand washing and breastfeeding, have sharply lowered child mortality across the globe. The vast majority of the world's newborns are now immunized against diseases such as measles, polio, and yellow fever, and the widespread use of oral rehydration salts has made cholera deaths increasingly rare.[13] According to the World Bank, infant mortality decreased by half between 1960 and 2005 in 80 percent of the countries for which there are data, and global average life expectancy increased from thirty-one years in 1900 to almost sixty-nine years by 2009.[14]

Extending lives is, of course, a good thing. Preventing avoidable death and infirmity and affording people the opportunity to lead productive lives is the raison d'etre of global health. The problem is that although life expectancies for the poor have increased in low- and middle-income countries, they have done so without the gains in personal wealth and better health systems that accompanied the rise in longevity in most developed countries.[15] With the significant exception of China, the poor have not benefited from the recent economic growth in developing countries. The number of people living on less than $2 per day has remained around 2.5 billion since 1981.[16] Income disparities have increased. More than 70 percent of the world's poorest people now live in middle-income countries.[17] Meanwhile, health-care spending, although slowly expanding in Latin America, the Middle East, and parts of Asia, remains incredibly low.[18] The state of Connecticut spends more on health than the thirty-eight low-income countries in Sub-Saharan Africa combined.[19]

While childhood and communicable diseases are on the decline worldwide, malnutrition and tuberculosis, water- and vector-borne diseases, and HIV/AIDS remain problems in the poorest developing countries, in Sub-Saharan Africa and South Asia in particular.[20] With little public support and facing this double burden of disease, the poor in developing nations often cannot afford preventive or chronic care, increasing the odds of disability and death from diabetes, cancer, and other NCDs that people contract after their adolescent years.

The nearly nonexistent regulation of tobacco, alcohol, and processed food products in many developing countries compounds the challenges of rampant poverty and inadequate health care by increasing the likelihood that poor people will develop NCDs. Governments lack accountability to their constituents for the consumption of products for which the health consequences are not apparent for years. Regulators face strident opposition from foreign and local tobacco, food, and alcohol producers—some of which may be fully or partly owned by the government. Governments fear that increased taxes on unhealthy products will harm local economic interests and incite political unrest. Consumers in many developing countries are not fully aware of the health consequences of tobacco and processed foods. Patient groups are nonexistent or a minor presence in most developing countries. Civil litigation, which has played a critical role in improving tobacco control and education in the United States, is far less common and successful in developing countries.[21] Inadequate labeling and regulation of ingredients hurt the poor most, since they have neither the opportunity to educate themselves about health risks nor the money to buy healthier food.[22]

Meanwhile, freer trade and the increased global integration of tobacco, food, and beverage markets are overwhelming the little public health infrastructure that does exist in many developing countries. Developing countries that represent relatively small commercial markets have limited ability to demand labeling and content changes in order to reflect local needs to food, alcohol, and tobacco products produced for global consumption. Multinational corporations may be better resourced than the governments seeking to oversee them. With stagnating sales in high-income nations, multinational companies now target low- and middle-income countries, using sophisticated advertising campaigns and trade initiatives to drive growth.

Tobacco companies, in particular, use billboards, cartoon characters, music sponsorships, and other methods now prohibited in most of the developed world to entice women, who used to be less likely to smoke than men.[23] Multinational tobacco companies dispute resolution under trade and investment agreements to block restrictions on these advertising and labeling practices.[24] These tactics have raised tobacco sales across Asia, Eastern Europe, and Latin America, and many expect them to do so in Africa. Between 1970 and 2000, cigarette consumption tripled in developing countries.[25] In more than 60 percent of the countries surveyed in a 2008 study by WHO and the U.S. Centers for Disease Control and Prevention (CDC), girls now smoke just as often as boys.[26]

Low- and middle-income countries are urbanizing at a rate unprecedented in human history. It required fifty years for the world's urban population to increase from 220 million to 732 million in 1950. By 2008, more than half of the global population lived in urban environments and the world's urban population is expected to reach almost 5 billion (60 percent) by 2030.[27] The vast majority of this urbanization is occurring in low- and middle-income countries. China and India have the largest urban populations; cities in Africa and South Asia are growing the fastest.[28] Urbanization is particularly pronounced in formerly small- and medium-sized cities in developing countries with limited public health infrastructure.[29] The result has been slums—90 percent of which are now in developing countries and house nearly 1 billion people.[30] The inhabitants of these densely packed areas, faced with pollution outdoors and the burning of fuels indoors, are more susceptible to cardiovascular and respiratory diseases. Slum dwellers are more likely to buy tobacco products and cheap processed foods and less likely to have access to adequate nutrition or public health education.

The NCD Epidemic in Developing Countries

NCDs are increasing faster in low- and middle-income countries; arising in younger, working-age populations; and having much poorer health outcomes than seen in developed countries. This challenge has arisen from increased longevity without the improved living conditions, better nutrition, and gains in wealth that accompanied aging in most developed countries decades ago. Urbanization and changes in global trade are accelerating and exacerbating these problems.

NCDs are increasing even more rapidly in low- and middle-income countries than originally predicted. According to WHO, 80 percent of deaths from NCDs now occur in low- and middle-income countries, up from 40 percent in 1990.[31] WHO projects cancer incidence to increase by 70 percent in middle-income countries and 82 percent in lower-income countries by 2030.[32] If current trends persist, the World Bank reports that the number of people over forty in China with at least one NCD could double or triple over next two decades.[33]

NCDs in emerging-market nations are also arising in young working-age populations at higher rates and with more detrimental outcomes than in wealthy states. People with NCDs in middle-income countries are more than twice as likely to die before age sixty as those in high-income nations, and people in low-income countries are four times as likely to do so. Ninety percent of the 9 million premature deaths from NCDs in 2010 occurred in low- and middle-income countries.[34]

NCDs that are preventable or treatable in developed countries are often death sentences in the developing world. Whereas cervical cancer can largely be prevented in developed countries thanks to the human papillomavirus (HPV) vaccine, in Sub-Saharan Africa and South Asia it is the leading cause of death from cancer among women.[35] With early diagnosis and the widespread availability of insulin, deaths from juvenile diabetes in high-income countries are rare; low- and middle-income countries experience over 80 percent of diabetes deaths worldwide and virtually all of the deaths from juvenile diabetes.[36] Ninety percent of children with leukemia in high-income countries can be cured, but 90 percent of those with that disease in the world's twenty-five poorest countries die from it.[37] The mortality rate in China from stroke is four to six times as high as in France, Japan, or the United States.[38] Almost 90 percent of chronic obstructive respiratory deaths worldwide occur in low- and middle-income countries.[39] By 2030, NCDs will be the leading cause of death and disability in every region of the world, including Africa.[40]

The rise of NCDs has devastating social and economic consequences for developing countries. Early onset of already chronic illnesses consumes scarce health-care resources and undermines the capacity of developing country health systems to respond to infectious and nutritional diseases and other health threats.[41] The toll of NCDs on the young and middle-aged consumes household budgets and robs families of their primary wage earners.[42] NCDs sap worker productivity, undermine economic development, and perpetuate the cycle of poverty, insecurity, and infirmity in the communities in which these diseases are most endemic in low- and middle-income countries.[43] A recent report by Harvard University and the WEF projects that over the next two decades, NCDs will inflict $14 trillion in economic losses on the developing world.[44]

The Right Prescription

Focusing on the global burden of all NCDs generally generates headline-sized estimates of the economic costs and death and disability connected with these diseases, but not the consensus, popular and donor support, and coherent policies needed to make progress on behalf of the patients with greatest need. Greater prioritization is needed. The international community should focus on the NCDs and risk factors especially prevalent among the developing country poor and on the particular needs of their governments to address them. This more targeted approach would allow initiatives to build international support needed for concrete prevention and control measures and to help isolate the potential opponents to effective action.

International efforts on NCDs should not and need not seek to replicate the recent global health initiatives on HIV/AIDS, malaria, and other infectious diseases. The solutions needed for NCDs do not require mobilizing massive resources to purchase and distribute life-saving technology. The measures necessary to prevent NCDs in healthy people are well known, and affordable medicines exist for improving care for those already living with these diseases. The World Bank estimates that developing countries could lower their projected rates of disability and death from NCDs by half by raising taxes on and restricting the marketing of tobacco and alcohol, reducing salt and trans fats in foods, and using beta-blockers, aspirin, and other low-cost interventions to control hypertension.[45] Treatments for NCDs, such as insulin and asthma inhalers, are no longer under patent and would do much to reduce avoidable disability and death if made more widely available.[46]

The challenge in many developing countries is that implementation of these NCD programs must be accomplished in the midst of dramatic demographic changes and strident industry opposition, and without the regulatory and health infrastructure, expertise, and capacity present in developed countries. With international support, however, progress can be made with the same tactics used in many other global health efforts prior to recent international efforts on HIV/AIDS. These tactics include: (a) generating the evidence and technical consensus on solutions required in the settings of need; (b) reducing those solutions into an implementable technical package and providing technical support, as needed, to local officials on their implementation; (c) improving the country-level accountability for the implementation of that package with international surveillance and in-country civil society support; and (d) ensuring adequate and predictable funding, where needed, for these efforts. As described by Ruth Levine in her 2004 book *Millions Saved*, these tactics have been behind many of the greatest successes in global health over the last thirty years.[47]

International tobacco control would be a good place to start. Few global health threats can compare with the human and economic toll of tobacco-related diseases in developing countries. Tobacco use kills more people annually than HIV/AIDS, tuberculosis, and malaria combined and is projected to disable and kill hundreds of millions more in the coming decades, mostly in low- and middle-income countries.[48]

Tobacco use is the only leading risk factor common to all the major disease groups of NCDs: cancer, diabetes, cardiovascular, and respiratory disease.[49] The scientific consensus that tobacco use and second-hand smoke cause a plague of terminal and disabling diseases no longer faces serious challenge. By increasing support for tobacco control in developing countries, the international community could help reduce one of the most significant threats to global health today.

Fortunately, a platform for combating tobacco use already exists: the WHO Framework Convention on Tobacco Control (FCTC), a binding treaty with 173 Member States that mandates taxes, advertising, and other measures to lower demand for tobacco products.[50] WHO, in partnership with Bloomberg Philanthropies, developed a package of evidence-based strategies, called MPOWER, to turn the broad mandates of the FCTC into practical programs that developing-country governments can implement.[51] Together with the CDC and Canadian Public Health Association, WHO tracks global tobacco use and the implementation of the FCTC and publishes the results in a biennial report.[52] The Campaign for Tobacco-Free Kids and other organizations work with local media and civil society to hold governments accountable for enforcing the recommendations put forth by MPOWER.

International tobacco control programs are making progress, but they are limited by a lack of funding and technical capacity within developing countries, as well as fierce industry opposition. Outside the handful of developing countries that receive support from Bloomberg Philanthropies and the Bill and Melinda Gates Foundation, tobacco control in developing countries remains woefully underfunded.[53] A low-cost way to extend anti-tobacco programs to other developing countries is for the international community to integrate these programs into existing global health initiatives on tuberculosis and maternal and child health. Tobacco excise taxes and cigarette-package labeling have proven to be among the most effective at cutting tobacco use prevalence, but their implementation in developing countries at WHO-recommended levels has lagged. Countries with experienced tobacco tax and regulatory authorities should increase their mandates and resources to support the efforts of their developing country counterparts. Developed countries must also stop trying to reduce tobacco tariffs and protect tobacco-related investments in their trade agreements with low-income nations.[54] With these affordable measures, developed countries can do much to support the world's poorest countries in their efforts to make sustainable progress against tobacco use.

Meanwhile, international initiatives to reduce the intake of alcohol, trans fats, and salt should focus for the time being on country-level programs and industry partnerships. While tobacco products cannot be made healthful, the same is not true for alcohol, food, and beverage products that can be healthful with appropriate ingredients, adequate labeling, education, and moderation. Partnerships with these producers and retailers can be productive and help reduce opposition to progress. The voluntary salt and fat reductions adopted by PepsiCo across its product lines stand out as a positive example. These voluntary measures may not replace the long-term need for taxes and regulations in these areas, but they could promote progress until the capacity and popular support for such programs grows. When that time comes, the improvements made in country-level regulatory and taxation systems for tobacco control could be extended to address alcohol, trans fats, salt, and other NCD risk factors. Integrating the monitoring of alcohol and unhealthy food consumption into the existing international tobacco-surveillance system would also offer a cost-effective means of collecting evidence on the implementation of the initiatives in these areas.

Yet prevention measures alone cannot solve the NCD problem. Effective therapies already exist for many NCDs—insulin, asthma inhalers, and beta-blockers and other hypertensive medications—and are off-patent, but remain unavailable or inappropriate for use in many low- and middle-income settings. Expanding existing international and regional vaccine procurement mechanisms to include essential NCD medicines would help developing countries get the prices and predictable supplies they need to meet the needs of their citizens. More donor support is needed for product development partnerships, such as PATH, which are working to adapt existing medical technologies such as diabetes diagnostics and HPV vaccines for NCDs for low-income country use.

Finally, the international community should not forget the poorest countries, where the consumption of unhealthy products is low and tobacco-prevention programs would offer only limited benefits to those suffering from cancer, diabetes, and other NCDs. Increased aid is needed to address NCD treatment needs in the poorest countries, such as the Sub-Saharan African countries in which Partners in Health and other organizations are helping treat cancers.[55] When and where appropriate, these international NCD efforts should harness existing treatment platforms in these countries, such as those established by the U.S. President's Emergency Plan for AIDS Relief (PEPFAR) to lower the costs and increase the reach of these treatment programs.

From Village to Slum

Global health needs are changing. The NCD crisis in developing countries is representative of a set of emerging health challenges— environmental pollution, food safety, urban sanitation, substandard medicines, and road safety and other injury prevention—that have begun to dominate the global burden of disease. These other challenges share similar origins as NCDs—freer trade, unprecedented urbanization, and limited local government capacity—and likewise have devastating consequences for the world's poor. The complexity of these global health challenges and their existence in rich and poor countries alike are testing, however, the convictions and ingenuity of a donor and policy community traditionally motivated by charity, self-interest, and the potential for simple, technological interventions.

Moving forward will require a renewed and sustained commitment from the international community to reducing the avoidable deaths and infirmity that result from persistent poverty and inequity. The same commitment motivated global health initiatives on infectious diseases and maternal and child health, and should do so again with regard to NCDs and the other emerging challenges in this new era of global health. Because that commitment will depend on prioritization and humility among the global health community, promoting every shared public health concern as a global problem with implications for economic development and national security will merely dissipate the urgency on genuine global health challenges.

Progress on NCDs and these other emerging global health challenges also will require different tools. Past global health initiatives have been primarily devoted to delivering food, drugs, and other health technologies to the world's poor. It was possible to achieve progress in environments with dysfunctional government. It is not possible to adopt and enforce effective regulation on smoke-free public places, food and drug safety, urban sanitation, and road traffic in such settings. Accordingly, the fundamental challenge in this new era of global health will be governance, more so than new medicines.

Meeting this challenge will require a recalibration of global health resources. Philanthropic foundations, international surveillance, and technical agencies, like the CDC, will play an even more dominant role in global health initiatives. The contributions of diplomatic and aid institutions, such as the U.S. State Department and the U.S. Agency for International Development, will remain important, but they will be limited to funding pilot programs and creating the international consensus that can give the governments of emerging-market nations courage in the face of industry opposition. Closer collaboration between trade and regulatory officials, like the Office of the U.S. Trade Representative and the U.S. Food and Drug Administration, on international standards could make it easier for developing countries to adopt strict tobacco, food, and drug regulations that would facilitate both commerce and public health. More support will be needed for the cash-strapped WHO, which takes on global health issues that others will not. Initiatives against NCDs and these other emerging health challenges should be coordinated on regional platforms, with the WHO and regional entities such as the Pan American Health Organization, which convene states with similar cultures, economic circumstances, and demographic challenges. With these low-cost measures, the international community can extend the same lifesaving support that it has provided to the little boy in a rural, dusty village to the working-age woman living in an urban slum.

Humanitarian Response in the Era of Global Mobile Information Technology

VALERIE AMOS

Technology is among the most difficult topics to tackle in a chapter designed to be relevant for more than a few months. The digital revolution has brought, and is still bringing, many positive changes to the world. In the humanitarian sector, technology has revitalized worldwide volunteerism through crowd-sourcing, driving closer cooperation between the humanitarian and the for-profit sectors. It has empowered people who receive humanitarian aid and improved the way we manage information.

These changes have challenged old assumptions and reshaped existing systems in deep and unexpected ways. In this chapter, I will set out what new technology offers us across the humanitarian sector; highlight the mutual benefits of the sector's newly formed relationship with the technology sector; and suggest how we can improve the partnerships we are building to tap the full potential of information technology in our work.

Building Resilience

The first step in crisis response starts well before disaster hits. Developing resilient early warning systems helps communities withstand even major hazards. Mobile technologies offer improved ways of doing this.

Social and economic data, including maps, are essential to building resilient communities. Most conversations about public safety and assistance take place around a map. Mobile technology enables us to compile, share, and update maps more quickly and accurately than ever before, so that we can put our resources where they will be most effective, at both local and national levels.

The Grassroots Mapping Project (www.grassrootsmapping.org) uses inexpensive techniques, like balloons and kites, to compile maps that are aimed at changing how people see the world in environmental, social, and political terms. The organization worked in the New Orleans area in 2010 to map the BP oil spill, and is now broadening its scope to explore inexpensive and community-led means to measure and explore environmental and social issues.

Interactive mobile technology can also enhance the ways maps are used, making them a valuable tool for advocacy and development—crucial elements of building resilience. In Somalia, the Danish Refugee Council (DRC) is running an online map of its development projects in rural areas. The map shows every village with a project funded by the DRC. Clicking on a village reveals details about the project, its aims, and its progress. Somalis in the diaspora have started to use the map to decide on the best villages for their donations. These diaspora communities are even topping up the original funding offered by the DRC—an unexpected side-effect of the project.

Interactive mapping has been taken up at the international level by the World Bank, which launched the Mapping for Results platform in October 2010. This initiative visualizes the location of World Bank projects and enables citizens and other stakeholders to provide direct feedback, enhancing the transparency and social accountability of these projects.

For select countries, the platform provides not only geographic information about World Bank-financed programs, but also allows users to overlay disaggregated poverty, population density, and human development data (i.e., infant mortality rates, malnutrition, etc.). Population density is available for 107 countries; data on mortality, maternal health, and malnutrition data are available for forty-three countries; and poverty data for thirty-one countries. Such moves toward transparency will undoubtedly have implications for funding and development in the future.

Mobile cash transfer programs, which deliver vouchers or cash directly to recipients, can also play a crucial part in building resilient communities, help people to withstand slow-onset crises, and build sustainable livelihoods. Programs can be integrated with national social security systems to maximize impact. As in so many areas, humanitarians are only beginning to investigate the possibilities that this technology offers.

Local Action

In all disasters, local communities form the front line of the crisis response. If local people have access to cutting-edge technology during an emergency, they can be extremely effective in communicating the needs of affected communities to each other and to local, regional, and international aid organizations.

The formation of local social networks to spread news, including tips and warnings about impending weather events or volcanic activity, is another important way in which mobile technology has contributed to disaster prevention and recovery. These tools are increasingly being used in disaster-prone areas. For example, civil authorities in Mexico City have recently rolled out a free mobile application that will warn people when an earthquake is imminent. The application triggers an alarm on the phone once an earthquake of magnitude 6.5 or higher has been detected. During the 2010 eruption of Mount Merapi outside Jogjakarta in Indonesia, a local communications group called Jalin Merapi used Twitter, Facebook, SMS, and local radio to keep the community informed in real time and to understand and communicate emerging needs.

Local film makers in Thailand also used digital technology to spread the word during a flood emergency in 2011. They posted a series of ten videos on YouTube aimed at bringing home to people the seriousness of the situation. In one, they represented the billions of cubic meters of water bearing down on Bangkok as an equivalent volume of blue whales. The main video in the series has been viewed more than a million times.

Looking to the future, it is clear that local mobile networks also have much to offer in disseminating information during a crisis. The response to a tornado that hit the town of Joplin in Missouri in May 2011 was partly coordinated through a Facebook page. The page, Joplin Tornado Information, was set up within two hours of the tornado striking and began connecting needs, resources, transportation, and storage requirements. It soon had nearly 50,000 fans. Relief organizations, churches, and news sources started to post information on the page, including the news that water trucks had arrived in the town.

Similarly, social media was a primary source of communication after an earthquake and tsunami struck northern Japan in March 2011. Within an hour of the earthquake, an estimated 1,200 tweets per minute including references to the disaster were being posted on Twitter. Many Japanese people used Facebook, Twitter, and the Japan-specific site Mixi to share information and keep in touch. These examples from highly connected countries with robust infrastructure show what will be possible in an increasing number of countries in future.

Many of the most useful new mobile platforms are also accessible to locally based groups and even those affected by crises. For example, Crowdmap (www.crowdmap.com) allows anyone to set up a mapping project on the Ushahidi platform (www.ushahidi.com), a tool to crowdsource information using multiple channels. This technology has recently been used by people in Syria to track unrest there in real time.

Early Warning

Information saves lives, and the UN is heavily investing in global systems to alert early responders in the event of a major sudden-onset crisis like an earthquake or typhoon. The UN Office for the Coordination of Humanitarian Affairs (OCHA) runs a web-based real-time information channel for affected countries and bilateral responders used immediately after major disasters. This channel, known as the Virtual On-Site Operations Coordination Centre (OSOCC) is used by most Member States and regional organizations. Since 2004, the Virtual OSOCC has been part of the Global Disaster Alert and Coordination

System (GDACS), which is an international network of disaster information systems aimed at facilitating information exchange and coordination in the first hours after a natural disaster. GDACS includes an automatic disaster alert and notification system, as well as automatic feeds of related disaster maps and satellite images. GDACS alerts are submitted to subscribers by e-mail and SMS text message minutes after disaster events to inform about the possible humanitarian impact of disasters.

A major initiative in this area is the UN Global Pulse, which was created by UN Secretary-General Ban Ki-moon in 2009 to explore opportunities to use real-time data to gain a more accurate understanding of well-being, and assess levels of stress, particularly on vulnerable people. Global Pulse tracks the human impacts of crises as they happen, and enables the UN to access feedback in real time on how well its responses are working.

The strategy has three interdependent areas of activity: "Data Research" to assess community well-being; a "Technology Toolkit" of free and open source software tools so development experts can mine data, share ideas, and make evidence-based decisions; and the "Pulse Lab Network," an integrated network of country-level innovation centers, bringing together government experts, UN agencies, academia, and the private sector to apply new applications of data to development challenges. Global mobile communications technology plays a crucial role in all these areas.

Global Pulse stresses the importance of creating actionable information, that is, policy recommendations, from raw data. The project detects what it calls "digital smoke signals" that indicate changing conditions and behavior. For example, if people start to reduce unnecessary expenses and sell off property and livestock, this is an early predictor of food insecurity and malnutrition. The initiative's main technology tool is a social network called Hunchworks, which helps experts share hypotheses, collect evidence, and make decisions.

In addition to this major international push, national and regional disaster management agencies also recognize the importance of using mobile technology in early warning systems. Social media was used widely during the January 2012 floods in the Philippines, which has the fifth-largest number of Facebook users in the world. Some 130,000 people made use of the government's Weather Watch website to receive updates on conditions for travel by road and sea. The site issued warnings on collapsed roads and dangerous sea conditions for fishermen. Many Filipinos who lack access to computers used their smart phones to receive this information.

Saving Lives in Crisis: An Evolving Picture

The scope for technology to help emergency responders was first explored after the magnitude 7.0 earthquake that hit Port-au-Prince, Haiti, in January 2010. With hundreds of thousands of people dead and more than a million homeless, governments pledged hundreds of millions of dollars, but ordinary citizens also contributed enormous amounts of money. Much of this was raised through mobile phone text messages, marking the dawn of a new era of instant electronic donation.

Amid the chaos, one utility was up and running within days: the mobile phone network. Over the previous five years, Haiti had undergone a transformation. Two mobile phone networks run by Digicel and Voila covered almost the entire country. These networks had become the country's leading industry. Haiti in 2010 was the poorest country in the Americas, but its people could communicate with each other, and with the world, even after the earthquake. This meant that they could share information via local and international radio and online networks and participate in online mapping projects.

Volunteers gathered online to look for ways to communicate with Haitians and map the crisis, using a raft of innovative tools from SMS messages to collaborative mapping platforms and systems to mine data from social media sites like Twitter. Within hours of the earthquake, the collaborative mapping platform Ushahidi set up a site to collate and map data from text messages, social media, official situation reports, and other sources of information.

An SMS short code, 4636, was established with Digicel for local people to send and receive emergency-related messages. (Short codes work like the emergency numbers 911 or 999 as easily memorized shorthand for longer 'traditional' numbers.)

OpenStreetMap,[1] a collaborative system to mark names and key points on a publicly available online map, started charting the transformed city of Port-au-Prince; this became a vital resource for aid responders. A Haitian OpenStreetMap team formed a close relationship with the International Organization for Migration and their work informed the entire aid effort.

All these steps produced an incremental change in attitudes toward the use of mobile technology in a disaster zone and this had a significant impact during the Libya crisis of early 2011. Part of the challenge in Libya was that the UN did not have physical access to much of the country and was struggling to get a clear picture of what was happening. Although there was data available online, there was no way to verify and process this information. The Standby Task Force (SBTF)—a self-organized group of volunteers born from the Haiti experience—responded by creating the Libya Crisis Map.[2] The map worked by collating data from dedicated collaborators and the general public to plot incidents or trends, such as refugee flows, on a map in real time. A UN specialist reviewed the data, looked for patterns, and found ways to use this information.

Another significant step forward came during the largest humanitarian crisis of 2011: a massive regional drought in eastern Africa. The United Nations High Commissioner for Refugees (UNHCR) approached the SBTF which activated a network of volunteers to analyze thousands of images and chart settlements, tagging over a quarter of a million features.[3] This helped to identify newly built urban areas and to get a better picture of the numbers there who needed help.

Mobile Phones Change the Game: Two-Way Communication and Electronic Cash

The spread of cheap communications technology also promises to change the entire aid model fundamentally by changing the relationship between humanitarian workers and those affected by emergencies and disasters. A 2011 study by the U.S.-government-funded Internews Media Support NGO examined the experience of Somalis in the world's largest refugee camp in Dadaab, Kenya, and found that establishing two-way communication with affected communities was not a high priority for aid workers:

> Serious communications gaps between the humanitarian sector and refugees . . . are increasing refugee suffering and putting lives at risk. . . .
> . . . large numbers of refugees don't have the information they need to access basic aid; more than 70 per cent of newly-arrived refugees say they lack information on how to register for aid, and similar numbers say they need information on how to locate missing family members.[4]

Some aid organizations have begun to contact affected communities using communications technology. The International Federation of Red Cross and Red Crescent Societies (IFRC) is aiming to set up formal agreements with mobile phone providers in fifty disaster-prone countries. They will be able to see how many people are connected to each telephone aerial, and send out mass text messages. These could be carefully targeted in the case of localized flooding, or used for early warning of hurricanes or other adverse weather events. The connection could also be used to seek feedback on crisis conditions in an area, or even to locate people trapped under rubble.

Another development that will have a significant impact on the relationship between donors, humanitarians, and affected communities is the rise of mobile electronic cash. This has the potential to transform the humanitarian sector through direct transfers to large numbers of people affected by emergencies and through targeted transfers to individuals to conduct specific tasks, including monitoring, assessments, purchasing medicines for a clinic, and so on.

In crisis after crisis, markets have been shown to provide supplies extremely quickly. The problem is that the most vulnerable people can not afford to buy anything. Instead of meeting this shortfall with huge, expensive international logistics chains that undercut the market, the advocates of mobile cash transfers argue that it is cheaper and more effective to provide vulnerable people with money or vouchers to buy what they need.

This proposition is fraught with controversy. Transferring cash creates many logistical challenges, and will not always provide what is most badly needed. The World Food Programme (WFP) says it chooses which kind of aid will be most appropriate depending on various factors, including cost-effectiveness and availability of food. "When appropriate," it states, "cash and vouchers can meet more closely the needs of targeted vulnerable people."[5]

Several programs are already using electronic money and vouchers. In 2009, the WFP launched a mobile delivery and tracking system based on electronic vouchers in Zambia, redeemable through mobile phones thanks to a technology platform provided by Mobile Transactions Zambia. Recipients registered by uploading a national registration card into the system. They then received a scratch card that they could redeem at specific vendors.

A program in Niger in West Africa shows that this technology has potential even where mobile phone ownership is low. In 2010, the international NGO Concern joined forces with the mobile network operator Airtel to facilitate mobile money transfer to 4,000 households affected by drought-related food insecurity, in an attempt to reduce operating costs and increase benefits to recipients. Other households received cash in envelopes. Concern partnered with Tufts University to investigate the impact of the mobile money transfer. They found that receiving mobile money saved time for recipients, who did not have to walk to a distribution point or wait for a delivery. The mobile money recipients also bought a greater variety of food types and nonfood items and grew a wider variety of crops; the reasons for this were not clear. Even illiterate households had no problem accessing the money; they sought help from relatives and neighbors.

Private Sector Involvement

Another element of this changing landscape is the growing interaction between the aid sector and the private sector. This interaction has brought the energy and financial power of the private sector to benefit humanitarian causes. It has also benefited the private sector, with a growing acknowledgment from companies that encouraging healthy societies provides many tangible and intangible benefits.

After the Haiti earthquake, one of the country's mobile phone providers, Digicel, provided its 2 million customers with $5 of free credit, which enabled them to get in touch with each other and the outside world, and build a better picture of the situation at the height of the crisis. Digicel also donated generators, phones, and credit to fifteen radio stations in Port-au-Prince to help them reach their listeners. This provided an essential conduit for humanitarian aid responders to get their message out to the general public.

Partnership with mobile phone providers also provided information on a grander scale in Haiti. A study by researchers from Sweden's Karolinska Institute and Columbia University[6] showed that it was possible to track the movement of displaced people by following their mobile phones. The study indicated that some 600,000 people had left the Haitian capital in the nineteen days after the earthquake, with clear implications for the provision of humanitarian aid. This tracking technology was also used after the Japanese earthquake and tsunami of 2011, and offers great possibilities for future emergencies, displacements, and epidemics, provided due attention is paid to privacy issues.

Partnerships between the UN and the private sector were initially philanthropic; the UN and partners would raise money from the private sector to fund projects which were often not related to the core business of the company in question. Today, these are genuine collaborations. An innovative partnership between the Vodafone Foundation and the UN Foundation known as the Technology Partnership has brokered relationships between UN agencies and some of the biggest companies in the world. WFP is working with partners including PepsiCo, Caterpillar, and Unilever. The IFRC has a long-running partnership agreement with Nestlé.

These partnerships reached a turning point when the technology sector began to make products cheap and robust enough to be relevant to the developing world. In December 2011, OCHA and Ericsson celebrated the 11th anniversary of their global partnership for the provision of GSM (Global System for Mobile Communications) and related services and expertise in support of humanitarian relief operations. Ericsson Response is the company's volunteer program that works to help OCHA in emergency situations by setting up mobile networks for voice and data communication. The team has been deployed fifteen times since 2001, most recently in Haiti in 2010, when its mobile network provided an average of 5,000 free calls per day to humanitarians for six months.

UNHCR, in partnership with Microsoft, is using communications technology to improve UNHCR operations and develop programs to help refugees rebuild their lives, store their data, and access new opportunities through education and connectivity. Microsoft supports UNHCR by providing technological expertise, while UNHCR contributes its fifty years of know-how in addressing challenging refugee issues. Google is working on several projects, including the improvement of financial tracking of donor contributions and is providing Google Earth services to some aid operations.

Private organizations contribute resources such as employee mobilization or secondment, funds, in-kind donations and expert services, cause-related marketing, and expertise to support humanitarian actors in relief and rehabilitation efforts. The private sector also brings leadership, assets, access to global networks, and a unique perspective that can greatly benefit our work.

For their part, companies are eager to partner when they add value. Working in the humanitarian sector provides a narrative which shows that they are making a sustained difference and builds a business case for their work, creating value for the company.

Ericsson says that their volunteer program empowers employees to make a difference in society and adds another dimension to employees' jobs, making them feel more motivated. In addition, the experience and knowledge gained through working in emergency situations enables them to develop resilient and sustainable technical solutions that will be relevant to their business in the longer term.

Both the humanitarian community and the private sector still have a lot to learn from each other. Companies have far more to offer than the aid sector is currently equipped to ask for. We know there are potential private sector partners who are struggling to understand the humanitarian system and how to play a part in it.

Overcoming Challenges: The Future

I see three main challenges to maximizing the value of new technology for aid work: defining and working with the physical limitations of the technology; transforming our institutional frameworks to take account of the changing environment; and dealing with cultural and even psychological barriers to the adoption of new working practices.

First, we need more experience and research to clarify concrete areas in which mobile technology offers significant benefits. One simple example is that in some cultures, mobile devices and computing power may be under the control of male heads of household, which could present problems in delivering messaging, information, or cash transfers to women or the elderly. Building trust in new financial instruments like cash transfers will be crucial to ensuring that they are taken up and used effectively.

There are also valid concerns about the "consumerization" of disaster communications, ranging from fears over what happens to user data in politically insecure environments to the proliferation of "white noise"—the paradox of being utterly overwhelmed with information but still unable to find the information needed for decision-making.

These efforts must take into account the need to mitigate the risks associated with ad hoc messaging in a disaster or a war zone, including managing expectations and avoiding any perception of political bias or putting in danger those that are highly vulnerable or at risk of political persecution. The technology must be used wisely if it is to be as effective as possible.

At an institutional level, the international community has built large and complex systems over the years to collate, analyze, distribute, and act upon information. These tend to be driven by experts, and organized hierarchically. Some of these structures are necessary and important to deal with issues of privacy, quality control, economies of scale, security, and political sensitivity. But working with new technology and new partners—including the new volunteer and technical communities, and those from the commercial sector—has demonstrated that these may be a barrier to full collaboration.

At a cultural and behavioral level, research has shown[7] that aid agencies typically perceive new technology as being expensive or difficult to use, requiring specialist knowledge and support. Senior managers can often be the most reluctant to embrace change as they may hold on to a traditional view of how programming should work. It will require vision and leadership to overcome this reluctance and move from the "pilot" phase to the wide-scale adoption of new technologies. Financial controllers must also be supportive in order for change to happen, and must be made aware that initial investments will yield efficiencies or cost savings over time.

A short chapter on such a rapidly evolving subject will inevitably leave out more than it contains and many of the specifics may quickly become out of date. However, it is possible to draw one conclusion that will stand the test of time. The uptake of new technologies is more than a technical phenomenon: it is essential to ensuring aid work is as effective and relevant as it needs to be.

Disasters and the Media

JEREMY TOYE

For the media, a disaster is not a tragedy. It is a challenge, an opportunity. A challenge for the traditional media to find out what is happening, how to get there, what is at stake, who is to blame. For the nontraditional media, the tweeters, Facebook friends, and bloggers, it is how to get the message out, who to include, when to re-tweet someone else's tweet. And for all of them, there is the chance to inform, to activate, or to enrage for a vast audience always turns to the media whenever a disaster strikes.

Those are some of the challenges, but there are opportunities too. It is not necessarily wrong, nor even cynical, for a decent journalist to see a disaster as an opportunity to get a good story. Journalists wept at the site of the Twin Towers falling, at Princess Diana's funeral. But they and their hard-pressed employers had a job to do, and in a disaster, no matter whether it's "natural" or "man-made," it gets harder but potentially more rewarding. And most media outlets will claim that they are there to serve noble ideals, that challenging authority and revealing the facts will lead to change for the better.

For the hard-bitten owners of commercial media, there is not only an opportunity to show expertise and concern for suffering but also a chance to revive flagging circulations and audiences.[1] In that large slice of the world where the state controls the media, it is a chance to show that government can move fast and help—unless, of course, it is the regime itself which is to blame for the disaster. For those among the millions of social media users who want to go beyond their circle of friends and what they had for breakfast, disasters spell a chance get help, to rally support, or to let their compassion or concern show through.

The media has traditionally been reactive to disaster. It has happened, so now let us surf the feelings of revulsion and compassion and maybe someone will do something about it. But the explosion of digital connectivity via instant satellite links, the social media and above all the cell phone is leading some to question whether the media should do something more about disasters *before* they happen: to educate, teach, and inform people in areas vulnerable to drought, famine, or flood; to build, plant, save water, stock grain, or practice first aid. While more traditional media may argue that their role is to present the facts and let others decide, social media opens the door for communities of all stripes to take charge of their destiny.

It is left to the readers, listeners, and viewers who turn to the media, in particular at times of disaster, to distinguish reality from rumor, fact from fiction, promotion from propaganda. To paraphrase the title of this book, is it more truth with less manipulation, or more noise with less clarity? Perhaps, More Heat than Light? In the middle of all this cacophony sits a wide variety of enterprises lumped together as "the Media" and (often friends, sometimes foes) the "aid professionals" whose role is not only to find out what's going on in what they may call a disaster-related scenario but also to do something about it.

Media and Disasters

Disasters have always been part of the media's staple diet, but in early times the dish was eaten cold. The eruption of Vesuvius in A.D. 79? By the time anyone had time to react, the elegant city of Pompeii was preserved in ash.[2] By the time of Lincoln's assassination in 1865, the invention and rapid expansion of the telegraph system meant the news spread across the United States in minutes.[3] Two world wars tested first print then broadcast journalism (and the extent that censorship would be tolerated), while advocates for change used media to move into the public glare. The suffragettes battling for votes for women, who chained themselves to London railings, calculated well that their photos would be used around the world.[4]

The Ethiopian famine of 1983–84[5] was a milestone in putting a remote human disaster into the living rooms of what used to be called the first world (as opposed to the third world, now more politely named the developing world). But even in the world's first TV war in Vietnam,[6] instant communication to the public and therefore instant reaction was rare because of limited technology and high expense. And there was still time for judicious editing along the way: the most gruesome scenes could be cut, prompting accusations of media manipulation and official sanitization.

CNN and the bombing of Baghdad bridged the technology gap to show the Iraqi capital as it was bombed. Then mobile telephony, webcams and YouTube matched technology with portability and minimal price. The death of Neda Agha-Soltan,[7] broadcast from a cell phone camera in an Iranian demonstration attacked by government forces, took the process to a point where the traditional media, in the sense of providing a link between event and audience, was almost redundant.

The events of the Arab Spring of 2011, though largely only disasters for the dictators forced out of power, showed that not only could you use the new media to inform the uninformed and marshal support, you could also tell your fellow demonstrators what was going on just a few meters away. And since there is a dark side to almost everything, security forces could monitor those same calls and sift through YouTube videos for the faces they could identify. A sinister side of social media was demonstrated in the UK riots in 2011[8] when rioters with no political agenda could use encrypted messaging to give news on which shops were ripe for looting. Blackberrys, so long seen as the smart tool for the wheelers and dealers of the commercial world, found a new, unwelcome market among gangs of youths who knew open SMS messages would be monitored by police. Huge numbers of passive security cameras recorded images of looters blithely trying on shoes.

Like a knife or an ax, media in the wrong hands can be a fearful weapon. The videotapes of Osama bin Laden fueled Al-Qaeda's campaigns and inspired its followers to further violence. As in the filming of journalist Daniel Pearl's killing in Karachi in 2002, instant communication was another weapon to be used to support a campaign.[9] Pearl's death was also a reminder that dozens of journalists have been killed in conflicts such as Iraq, Afghanistan, and Syria.[10]

No wonder, then, that much of the monitoring of social media and instant communications is being done by representatives of the more traditional media. Twitter feeds, recalling for wire-agency veterans like this author the brief Snaps and Bulletins used to alert media outlets to breaking news, could keep a single journalist in touch with a dozen places at once. Backed by two-way satellite communications and an array of gear, the BBC's man in Beirut, Jim Muir, could keep track of a host of Syrian cities under attack by the forces of a government that refused entry to anyone identified as a journalist.

While journalists on the frontline donned flak jackets to ride with rebel forces into Tripoli, others were scouring the airwaves in case Libyan leader Muammar Gaddafi should suddenly send an SMS message that he needed, say, sticking plasters. When he was found, his summary execution on screen[11] caused genuine shock, even in a world becoming inured to the blood and gore of battle. The execution was carried out by individuals in a remote place, but a cell phone camera made it a public event.

Natural disasters seem to happen most where access is least: an earthquake in the mountains of Pakistan; a tsunami from a quake deep below the Indian Ocean; drought and famine in one of Africa's most forbidding spots, Somalia. Yet even when a disaster happens in a country as sophisticated and accessible as Japan, and affects an industry as modern as nuclear power, the media is often hard pressed to get there. That being said, the single-minded determination of a journalist seeking out a story means that relief agencies often find that the media is alongside and even ahead of them.

No matter how reliable the firsthand source, no matter how venerated the wire services, every media outlet worth its salt wants its own staffer's byline, voice, or face to tell the story. And that costs money. Cut-price airfares suddenly fade away as affected airports close, helicopter hire soars like the machines themselves, and even the cost of a taxi will multiply if the driver thinks he might not be able to get back.

But for a while, some parts of the media seemed to have money to burn. The second half of the twentieth century saw a major expansion in the money spent gathering news of all kinds, especially disasters, and much of it was driven by television. The *Guardian* editor C.P. Scott could famously predict that "no good" would come of television,[12] but one of his rivals[13] in the UK's first commercial network could equally famously boast that he had been issued "a license to print money." The rival U.S. networks of NBC, CBS, and ABC could outbid each other in their coverage, each fronted by a household name, while CNN in unfashionable Atlanta endeavored to unseat them. The era of twenty-four-hour news channels had arrived, concentrating on breaking news whatever its actual significance. On quiet news days, they would play the same video or audio clip again and again. On the disaster days, they would swing into action, using prearranged links to a welter of broadcasters whose own styles have moved inexorably from studio sets to street scenes.

In the twenty-first century, mobile telephony has opened whole continents to information access like never before. African villages that may still have only one communal TV set now have smart phones. African populations have made an enormous leap across a technology spectrum that had offered them nothing before.[14] Contrast this with a few years ago when the headmistress of a large secondary school in Swaziland told this author her pupils had no idea where their World Food Programme (WFP) aid came from—"and neither do I."

With a little help, that headmistress could now show her pupils where the food comes from, tapping into smart phone links on YouTube, or running Skype chats with the people who might help them grow better crops themselves. Such access might encourage the donors to ask their "beneficiaries" what's required before they supply, and also combat the stultifying fatalism which leaves so many children just as stunted as their lack of vitamins. Media campaigns, such as the *Guardian*'s regular reports from the Ugandan village of Katine,[15] help that process, but real change may come when means of communication sit firmly in the hands of the villagers themselves. And that day is not far off as cell phones spread like wildfire across the world.

For many, information-overload led directly to compassion fatigue. A new drought in East Africa—or is it West Africa? (In fact, in 2011, it was both.) Urgent pleas for donations from a familiar group of agencies were met by an unusually slow response from Western governments battling budget cuts and fighting to maintain levels of aid pledged in rosier times. Members of the public gave generously, but there were legitimate questions about how many more times they would be asked to save the starving child. Proponents of development rather than emergency handouts trotted out the cliché that if you give a man a fish, he will eat for a day, if you teach a man to fish, you will feed him for life, to which a weary aid official responded: "Yes, but the lake's dried up . . ."[16] Templated stories gave the idea that disaster was recurrent, predictable, and followed patterns: from rubble to tented cities to cholera outbreaks to stories written on the first anniversary which so often begin with a child's name: "Muhammad lost half his family . . ."

With global financial turmoil gripping both the developed and developing worlds from 2008, the media could not escape a cold blast of reality. Famous titles disappeared from the newsstands as rising costs and falling audiences swamped them.[17] Equally famous names such as the BBC found financial support waning, forcing news teams from different divisions to work together to keep down costs. Advertising revenue, in particular for television and print, dropped away.[18] (Insurance costs alone could scupper the chances of sending a news team to cover an event that may or may not run into a major disaster.)

In some cases, the use of social media mirrored the agendas of the more familiar news outlets: delirious flattery for the latest music sensation, rage at a rape case, fervent support or ferocious condemnation of politicians like President Obama, who used the network brilliantly to help his election, and perhaps came to rue its impact on his ratings. At other times, the social network makes its own agenda. A thirty-minute video that attracted over 70 million online viewers in a week is a case in point. A small charity had a committed filmmaker produce a video on their work and on one of their targets—Joseph Kony.[19]

So it is no wonder that many branches of traditional media turn to cell phone screens, blogs, and onsite video channels to supplement and even substitute their own coverage. In one sense, they have been doing this for years: the international wire agencies[20] were the Twitters of their day, with largely anonymous correspondents filing reports from every capital and major city as wholesalers to the world's media retailers. They too have had to change their approach, providing elements of their coverage without charge on innumerable websites while charging premium rates for their very best material—most of it related to financial and commercial markets.

But disasters have a habit of echoing right through those trading floors, as carefully analyzed scenarios are turned upside down by events on the coast of Japan or in Haiti.

Disasters and Stakeholders

While the traders hit their keys in response to the latest disasters, a disparate set of groups spring into action. These are the "stakeholders," in the parlance of the aid world, who are thrown together whenever a disaster strikes:

- the government departments whose job it is to safeguard a nation's health, safety, security, and general well-being;

- the official international agencies, such as the United Nations (UN) humanitarian family, with global mandates to serve the vulnerable and dispossessed, backed by national and international funding; agencies such as USAID and Europe's ECHO;

- the myriad nongovernment organizations (NGOs), ranging from the Red Cross/Crescent and Bill Gates' Global Fund through religious charities to a couple of Texas carpenters building one home at a time for tsunami victims, all responding to the natural wave of sympathy and support that a disaster brings;

- communities, national, regional or local, who may be drawn from the victims of a disaster or from others threatened by it, or from generous people far away.

Almost all of them, in an emergency, will find themselves seeking the oxygen of publicity—or being sought out by a demanding media when they are already overwhelmed. How these groups use, and might better use, the media is a key factor in whether they emerge in the aftermath of disaster honored or ignored.

Stakeholders, Disasters, and the Media

Alistair Cooke, once the doyen of foreign correspondents with his weekly broadcast, *Letter from America*, remarked that the only way to judge a journalist was by the quality of his sources. Anyone in media hoping to present her readers, listeners, or viewers with a portrait of what is happening in the world of aid would make little headway without sources within the community of stakeholders. Some sources would be known to many, such as a minister or an agency head. Other sources may never show their faces in public—the "Deep Throat" of Watergate, the "usually informed" or "reliable" sources where trust lies more with the believing journalist than with the potentially opportunistic whistleblower.

How the potential sources among stakeholders interact with the media may not directly affect the work they do or should do. But how their supporters and critics see them, and how they react when asked for help or reject hindrance, can be influenced by how they are presented in the media.

Governments, Disasters, and the Media

When disaster strikes—either on a national or regional scale, or closer to home, say, within a government agency itself—is the time when a government's relationship to the media is put to the test. It may have to face international media if the crisis attracts global attention, but it is often at local and national levels that a good relationship with the local press pays off best.

Until the onset of social media, some governments could bask in the comfort of an entirely state-controlled media. They had little to fear from the Soviet-era *Pravda*, President Mubarak's fawning *Egyptian Gazette* or the broadcasts of Radio Peking under Mao Zedong. While a more open press has flourished in many countries since the fall of the Berlin Wall, radio and television, both with a wider reach, have remained a principal tool of dictators everywhere.

The products of such systems are invariably dull, pedantic, and so far removed from reality that even a disaster can be buried alive. Editorial staff who work under the yoke of malicious state control lose their perspective in their constant search for the ultrapositive. For the rest of the world, a lively, driven media may actually get read, heard, or seen—but it means their governments have to work harder to get a sympathetic hearing.

One of the first acts of any new government is to appoint an information minister. For journalists, alas, they rarely live up to their title.[21] The government spokesman (occasionally a woman, but more often than not, a man) usually has more to say, and, if they are truly professional, will always be ready to say it. But a journalist who relied on speaking only to spokespersons of any hue would have a lackluster career, because the spokespeople must invariably be "on message" and, if threatened, must guard the gates of government against assault.

Given half a chance, the spokesperson will attempt a more sophisticated role, that of "spin-doctor." Turning a nightmare catastrophe into a glorious triumph by becoming a spin-doctor is much resented by journalists, but there will always be those officials that cannot resist trying to put a positive spin on a clearly negative story. Another more mundane role of the spokesperson is equally important: they are a route to the top. Most journalists want to speak to the organ grinder, not the monkey, and they work hard to get the most senior voice they can. A friendly word with a spokesperson often works. This cozy relationship between the media and its principal sources may not look much like the bombast coming out of a dictator in front of his cowering head of broadcasting, but the aim is the same—to keep the message sweet.

In disasters beyond the control of government, events themselves will take precedence over the words of even the most powerful leader. But sooner or later the spotlight turns on who needs to fix the roads, drain the fields, house the homeless, and open the airports. Invariably it is government that finds itself in the limelight. For the journalists, the questions are easy: Why was help too slow or too rushed, why has so little or so much been spent, why wasn't this fixed last time, what's to stop it happening again?

Counterintuitively, the sooner those questions get posed, the easier they will be to answer. A good government mouthpiece should be out there immediately saying what is known so far. At that stage, few journalists will have their own information to challenge what is being said. But if the government waits "until the situation becomes clearer," chances are it will have become muddier. The spokesperson may now have some beautiful charts to show what has been done, but the enterprising journalist has been there, seen a different picture, and has the quotes and photos to challenge the official line.

It is at this point that officialdom starts to stonewall and denials multiply, not only of facts but of obvious conclusions.[22] Some spokespersons are very proud of being able to handle any question, no matter how tough. The trouble is they can look like a boxer who builds a great defensive shield but fails to land the punch that wins the bout. Some spokespersons defend so well that they rarely get around to saying anything positive about the organization that pays them so well.

Some are masters, however: the U.S. ambassador to the UN under George W. Bush, John Bolton, once declined to answer a tough question. When it was asked again in a different form, he said, "Go ahead, it will be interesting to see how many times you pose that question before you give up." It was Bolton, the archetypal neocon, who also said that you could chop ten floors off the top of the United Nations building in New York and "it wouldn't make a bit of difference."[23]

The UN, Disasters, and the Media

Lose ten floors off the UN HQ and a journalist might miss a couple of useful sources, but it is more likely to have a greater impact on the ground. When the UN Offices in Baghdad were bombed in 2003 it robbed the UN of sixty staff including its highly respected Iraq chief Sergio Vieira de Mello. Furthermore, it robbed journalists covering the conflict in Baghdad of the expertise, experience and data-gathering that makes the UN much sought-after by the media.

In times of disasters, journalists can rely on the UN for more than just quotes—for access, for vital statistics to back up their own anecdotal evidence, for protection if the story gets too hot. That is not to say that the UN is universally popular among journalists who often like to see themselves as much more in touch with events on the ground. It is quite easy to paint a picture of the UN as overpaid suits operating behind heavily protected walls, breezing around town in gleaming white Land Cruisers and ready to cut and run at the slightest hint of trouble.

What is undeniable is that the UN's hierarchical system of checking and rechecking can mean that its reports and responses take days to appear. It can also lead to heavy self-censorship to avoid upsetting the Member States who in the end own the UN—and some of whom themselves see the UN as the enemy within.

The United Nations Children's Fund (UNICEF) is widely judged by its sister agencies in the UN to be the most adept at news management. "They don't move without thinking about the media," grumbled a UN veteran who knows his agency has fewer media professionals worldwide than UNICEF has in one office. Another agency organizing a huge convoy into Iraq seethed when UNICEF turned up with a handful of trucks emblazoned with its name—and stole all the media thunder.

But one other reason why UNICEF is so well known—in spite of having an acronym whose original meaning is often forgotten[24]—is that it has National Committees. These organizations, independent of the agency itself and of each other, run much of the publicity and fundraising at the local level in many developed countries. Other agencies rely on their top executive to get their message across. Josette Sheeran came from a media background to head the WFP, and frankly, her glamorous appearance did no harm either.[25] UNICEF chief Carol Bellamy[26] may have been a tough taskmaster, but she could turn on the gritty charm for the media whenever required.

Increasingly, UN agencies are looking to the social media to go beyond their own circles to the public at large. Punchy blogs stripped of the UN's love for acronyms and words like "psychosocial" are posted within minutes of an event, as are emailed invitations to support a named child with a small donation.[27] Yet for many senior UN staff, releasing the genii from the social network bottle means losing control, and increased risk of stepping on the toes of their masters.

Some of those toes belong to the funding agencies, the donors whose decisions can make the difference between life and death in a disaster. For the UN and most other aid agencies, funding only flows in when a disaster strikes, the result of urgent appeals which make up so much of the early media coverage. But once funds start to arrive the UN teams on the ground are in the eye of the storm—and part of that storm is whipped up by another set of initials, the NGOs.

The NGOs, Disasters, and the Media

One UN agency counts over 1,100 NGOs as its partners. Though the term NGO might not be on everyone's lips, their individual names are among the world's best-known "brands"—the Red Cross and Red Crescent, World Vision, Oxfam, Save the Children, Greenpeace, Médecins Sans Frontières (MSF). And they are so well known because above all they know how to use the media.

The suffering child with huge eyes and a swollen belly is an enduring symbol of innumerable campaigns. Though glossy or homespun posters, charity workers shaking tins on street corners, and subsidized advertising play their part, it is the extent of media coverage which marks the successes from the also-rans. Public relations lore suggests that an unpaid article written by a real journalist is worth many times more than paid advertising space. The one-minute video promotions shown between TV bulletins may be fully sponsored, but an interview embedded in the bulletin itself will have a greater impact.

In disasters, television leads the way—and some of its material is made by the NGOs themselves. The high quality of even the smallest cameras, complete with realistic shaky images, means that broadcasters can show aid workers as they move in. NGO bloggers and tweeters have much more freedom than their UN counterparts not only to describe what they are doing, but to pin down those they feel should do more. MSF is renowned for calling everyone to task, lambasting all and sundry. The impact can be twofold—to prompt the slow-footed into action, and to raise funds from members of the public who admire their forthright manner—which in turn won MSF a Nobel Peace Prize.

As with the UN, NGOs are not universally popular. Their heavy guns sent into an emergency can shoulder aside their local colleagues and sour the work done in building good relations on the ground. Their solutions, worked out around a desk in a distant capital, might not gel with local communities who resist change. In their home countries NGOs are frequently questioned about how much of the funds they collect actually go to their beneficiaries and how much is spent on administration or travel.

And in all the turmoil of a disaster, the media is there looking over their shoulders. Once behind a lens a news photographer will stop at little to get the shot—and if there is a crowd, they will jostle along with their text counterparts. Like the UN, NGOs spend many hours training their staff to accept media as a necessity rather than a mere nuisance or an actual hindrance.

Some of the larger agencies try to ensure media coverage by taking selected journalists in with them. The journalists might insist on paying their way, and though they will be grateful for the access, the best of them will still keep their professional distance, and the wise trip organizer will keep a watchful eye in case the whole thing goes wrong.

Courting publicity for any cause can backfire. An aid worker in West Africa complained bitterly that a campaign to help people deliberately mutilated by rebel forces had turned sour when insistent photographers made them "into a freakshow," prompting revulsion rather than sympathy.[28] The maker of the Kony video mentioned earlier won notoriety himself when he was filmed running naked and in distress near his home.[29]

Providing access is only one of the ways an agile NGO can improve its media coverage. High-quality data-gathering pays off if boiled down to easily assimilated facts. Introductions to the main players or even something as simple as offering recorded samples of local music to a radio reporter yields dividends. Willingness to answer questions while providing graphic details on the importance and success of their work is the hallmark of an excellent NGO spokesperson—and they will be sought out wherever they land.

The Public, Disasters, and the Media

Journalists love to recount their adventures in getting to the scene of a disaster against insuperable odds. But even the most agile reporter cannot beat the victim of a catastrophe who pulls out a mobile phone, snaps a surprisingly high-quality shot, and sends it off around the world (even if in fact it was only meant for a faraway member of the family). Communities of such people have begun to exercise their advantages of local presence and knowledge to campaign on their own behalf.

Some communities use the NGO route, though it can be difficult to sort the genuine from the grifters.[30] The social media works well at the other end of the pipeline too. Email campaigns based on the old principle of chain-letters can raise large amounts of cash in very few days—though they too need careful scrutiny for scams and spams.

As the instant access of the social media spreads to every corner of the planet, the possibilities of community-inspired media getting ahead of a disaster are increasing. Rather than wait for a drought to hit, a well-organized community can launch a targeted appeal for money to buy grain, or sponsor wells, or agricultural extension work to identify more resilient crops. This puts powerful mitigating tools in the hands of those most affected.

Disasters and the Big Picture

Earthquakes, drought, floods, and fire have been with us since time began, and media of all types know about handling them. But what of the big-ticket items that worry so much of the world's thinkers and planners: climate change, environmental damage, deepening poverty, crippling disease, and the demand for universal education? If the media is adept at handling instant disasters, it is perhaps less assured in how to deal with these ongoing challenges. And while the media struggles, voices in the wings insist that it can do much more than report passively what it sees and hears.

All media, from the self-important "Thunderer" (as *The Times* of London once styled itself) to the humblest blogger, thrives on change. But they are also addicted to speed, and no matter how big the looming disaster of climate change, no matter how destructive rising poverty to the future of the global village, actual change can be very hard to spot and track day by day. Add a third motivator, which is controversy, and much of the media will struggle—to use an old print-era phrase—to "hold the front page!"

For example, it is well established that man-made climate change will have a catastrophic impact, but perhaps not for years to come. Polar ice melt will swamp whole island nations but is just an almost imperceptible drip-drip every day. The media might report the first findings and the most dramatic, but struggles to find the vital new "angle" it needs on a regular basis to avoid the unforgivable journalistic sin of running the same story twice. That the vast majority of the world's experts agree that man-made climate change is a huge threat and must be checked makes matters worse: Where is the opportunity for the "on the one hand, on the other hand" adversarial style of most established media?

No small wonder then that to the fury of the conventionally wise, the mavericks that decry climate change as "media hysteria" themselves become the ones who find journalists beating a path to their door.[31] Mix in the fact that media loves a rogue more than a saint, and "good causes" have a hill to climb. There is also a risk that well-meaning campaigners will "cry wolf," overstating their case in the interests of people who are genuinely suffering.

Concerns about life-threatening health risks fare better in the media. Bulletins from the World Health Organization about bird or swine flu are given huge publicity, which in turn drives governments to act fast.[32] Most journalists try hard to be careful with stories on the latest miracle cure for cancer, but it can be tough to separate hyperbole from reality when a highly respected agency or a world-famous actor is warning that an entire region is about to suffer the worst disaster it has ever faced.

Man-made disasters, principally wars, have an easier route to the front page. This time the old cliché that the first victim of war is Truth is difficult to avoid for the media and its sources alike. Like soldiers sending letters home from the front, almost all media will respect a degree of censorship in wartime—unless they are reporting for the other side, but then that tends to be called spying.

On the inside pages and in the TV and radio documentaries, there is a chance to take a more nuanced view of the long-term impact of a slow-burning threat, and many responsible media outlets do just that.[33] Plus, media outlets can hardly be blamed if the public prefers the celebrity scandal, the reality TV show or, enormously important for most media, the sport. So, can the media be more proactive in saving the planet, and can it ever be seen, as some would like, as "a Force for Good"?

Media: A Force for Good, Neutral, or a Necessary Evil?

Whenever media is in the dock—as it was after journalists at the Murdoch-owned *News of the World* in Britain were found to have hacked into the phones of a large number of its targets—the charges are familiar. It is intrusive, abusive, disrespectful, money-grabbing, salacious—and everyone knows that because they all read, see, and hear the media.

When a media house does a clear public service—the *Washington Post*'s exposure of Watergate, the *Sunday Times*' campaign on behalf of disfigured victims of the thalidomide drug—their achievement is honored by their jealous peers and grudgingly respected by the public. But since the media can only be judged by its latest story, the glory fades fast. Some media identify with carefully selected good causes, especially at festive times such as Christmas in Western countries.

Campaigners[34] argue that the media can do much more to educate and advise its audiences on critical issues affecting their lives. In the case of disasters, members of the public could be advised to stock certain types of food during periods threatened by drought, to erect flood defenses, to build stronger quake-proof houses, to boil drinking water, or to sleep under malaria-proof bed nets.

Along with every other communicator, the media cannot just say *useful* things. It must also say *interesting* things. Unlike a boss who can oblige a subordinate to read her demand to cut down on paperclips, the media cannot oblige anyone to look or listen to what they write or say. Journalists constantly look for new angles on old stories, but the burden also rests on their sources to make their material interesting, and not just important.

So, can media ever be neutral, a disinterested but by no means uninterested recorder of whatever happens? The unsung heroes (to this entirely biased writer) are the local, national, and international news agencies, the "wire services" who feed a constant flow of as-it-happens reports to almost all the world's established media, who then choose what they will use.

The blunt instrument of media can certainly be evil in the wrong hands. The radio stations in Rwanda that goaded and screamed the murdering gangs into genocide were using the same basic medium that Aung San Suu Kyi in Burma used to address her followers after years of government-imposed silence.[35] The walls of the Schindler's Factory museum in Poland display chilling Nazi newssheets alongside schoolgirl letters describing the devastating effects on their wartime lives.[36]

To get the most good out of media the campaigners for any cause must make what they say as persuasive and interesting as possible. Fortunately, there are some well-tried tools that help do the job.

Tools for Disasters

The dedicated media campaigner can tap into a range of tools that have long been used successfully to attract and maintain media attention, but first a word about *preparation*. "I have no idea what this interview is about" is an awful admission. A campaigner should use any encounter with the media as an opportunity to get across what is happening, what is being done and what is needed. Translating everything into the language of the café from that of the office is a vital step. Only then will the maximum benefit come.

The humble *press release* remains a staple of almost all aid agency media campaigns. It should be brief, tightly edited and contain all the salient facts, backed up by a powerful quote or two, and supplied with useful contact details. Thousands upon thousands hit the media every hour, and sadly most end up "spiked," in the bin.

A news release can be reworked as a series of *tweets*, a usable set of Q&As, or an *op-ed piece* penned by the most senior person available. But for maximum impact, a human being is required. And an *interview*, broadcast live, is still one of the best ways of getting the messages across. While it is more comfortable to chat with a reporter on the phone or (rare in these hectic times) over a beer or lunch, the journalist involved remains at liberty to select whatever elements he wants. A live interview reduces that risk dramatically, and a well-prepared and practiced interviewee will win out almost every time over even the most aggressive interrogator.

Once a journalist is "hooked," a *field trip* to a disaster area is a popular means of promoting a cause. Careful planning is essential, as is monitoring of results, as such trips are rarely cheap in financial terms and sometimes very expensive in terms of reputation.

Perhaps most risky of all is a poorly planned *news conference*, because if one journalist is a threat, a group of journalists is a radioactive hazard. Our advice at MediaTrain is to explore every aspect of media relations before resorting to a press conference, and then have it very firmly handled by a seasoned press officer who is not afraid to be a policeman for the day.

Whatever tools are used, they all need regular *polishing*. Practice interview technique in front of a mirror, write a new report in the alternative style of an op-ed piece, sit in on a press conference with the journalist's best-loved tool, a notebook. Many worry that too much practice can make messages sound overrehearsed and stilted: in this author's experience, the vast majority of people facing the media are far away from reaching that point in their media-facing lives.

Disasters and the Media: A Never-Ending Story

Whether a disaster is instant, such as an earthquake, or ongoing, such as climate change, the basic human urges to know what's going on, and to listen to a frightening story, will remain.

Whether the media transmits to the inside of your eyeball, or boils it all down to an entirely arbitrary 140 characters, or blasts it out of rows of loudspeakers no one can ignore, the awful, the terrible, the catastrophic will always be with us.

Though the media itself may never want to be a force for good (and sometimes wants to be deliberately evil), there are going to be well-meaning people who, with skill, speed, and ingenuity, can make the media a critical part of their toolbox. In turn, that may help prevent, predict or mitigate an impending disaster. Whatever happens, the media, in one form or another, will always be there to report it.

Toward a Culture of Safety and Resilience

IRINA BOKOVA

Disasters bring home the fragility of human societies. These events—I personally witnessed the devastation in Japan, Haiti, and Pakistan—remind us of the toll that natural disasters can have in the loss of life and infrastructure, setting development back for decades in some regions. In a context marked by rising incidences of disasters and worsening consequences, the rhythm of international cooperation should not be dictated by the pace of emergencies. Investing in disaster reduction and preparedness today is crucial to save lives and safeguard infrastructure tomorrow. At a time of limited means, it is a prudent investment and it is a smart investment. A dollar invested in disaster prevention can help save $5 to $10 in disaster response. The time has come for a paradigm shift—to shift emphasis away from solely relief and disaster response toward a culture of preparedness and prevention.

International cooperation in education, the sciences, culture, and communication and information has a vital role to play in building disaster resilient societies. We need to understand and anticipate risks. We need to train communities in first aid. We need to disseminate vital information. And in crisis situations, culture is more than a point of reference and a stabilizer—it is a foundation for reconstruction.

This is the role of the United Nations Educational, Scientific and Cultural Organization (UNESCO). It includes contributing to post-disaster situations. This might come as a surprise to those who think that education, science, and culture are long-term concerns, far from the imperatives of urgent humanitarian action. And yet UNESCO intervenes to prepare and support societies affected by conflict or disaster, guided by the conviction that education, the sciences, culture, and communication and information are "earthquake-proof standards" that are essential for resisting the shocks of the world today.

UNESCO was founded in the wake of World War II on the idea that peace had to be built on new foundations both between States and within them. Our 1945 Constitution opens with the memorable phrase: "Since war begins in the minds of men, it is in the minds of men that the defenses of peace must be constructed." Lasting peace could not be based solely on political and economic arrangements between States. It had to take roots inside societies, on the basis of mutual understanding.

This humanist vision was poignant in 1945. Today, worsening risks and diminishing resources make it all the more relevant. The resilience of societies must be built on more solid and more lasting foundations than just material and economic infrastructure. Human ingenuity is a powerful catalyst for disaster risk reduction.

Strengthening the Fabric of Societies

The frequency and intensity of disasters have increased in the last decade.[1] Often exacerbated by the effects of climate change, disasters create large humanitarian and development challenges. Population growth, urbanization, alteration of the natural environment, substandard dwellings and public buildings, inadequate infrastructure maintenance, global climate change, and grinding poverty—all of these exacerbate the risks and impacts of disasters. Studies of disaster trends suggest that each year 175 million children are likely to be affected by climate-related disasters alone. Moreover, approximately 875 million children live in high seismic zones and hundreds of millions are exposed to regular flooding, landslides, extreme winds, and fire hazards.

It is possible to prevent disasters, or at least to considerably reduce their effects, by strengthening the fabric of societies and by training local populations. Disasters result from the combination of an exposed, vulnerable, and ill-prepared population or community and a hazard event. The impacts can be devastating and varied. The tsunami of December 26, 2004, in the Indian Ocean—a region at the time with no warning system—caused the death of more than 200,000 people, compared to the 20,000 victims of the tsunami of March 11, 2011, in Japan, a country equipped with the most effective warning system in the world.

UNESCO works with national authorities and civil societies on the ground to make the case for education, culture, the sciences, and communication to be placed at the heart of all international efforts for disaster preparedness and conflict prevention. Throughout all of this we move in step with all members of the United Nations (UN) family. UNESCO plays a pivotal role in global collaboration for the understanding and assessment of natural hazards and the mitigation of their consequences, as well as the provision of post-disaster assistance. It is one of the principal partners in the global effort to mitigate disaster risks and forms part of the system of the United Nations International Strategy for Disaster Reduction (UNISDR).

In practice, UNESCO's action is guided by five major pillars. The first pillar consists in strengthening risk defense and anticipation systems. UNESCO works in the areas of earthquakes, landslides, volcanic eruptions, floods, tsunamis, and droughts with the mandate to help set up reliable early warning systems—such as the tsunami early warning systems coordinated by the Intergovernmental Oceanographic Commission (IOC) of UNESCO. UNESCO is working to create a flood defense scheme in the entire Indus valley in Pakistan. In the Horn of Africa, hit in 2011 by the worst drought in sixty years, UNESCO teams evaluate and locate underground water resources to limit the impact of the current crisis and prevent future crises. Activities also encompass the establishment of international and regional centers for the exchange and analysis of hazard and disaster data. For example, the International Platform for Reducing Earthquake Disasters, a network launched by UNESCO, builds on expertise gained by 1,300 seismologists and earthquake engineers in one hundred countries to ensure better preparedness against earthquakes. In the same spirit, UNESCO works to integrate disaster risk reduction into educational, cultural, and information systems.

The second pillar is to ensure the active participation of all populations concerned. There can be no resilience without the full involvement of individuals on the front line, trained to react rapidly and spontaneously to the worst-case scenario. No warning system can ever replace trained and educated communities. Everyone must be capable of rapidly analyzing a risky situation and making the right decisions. This can only be achieved if all individuals and societies are equipped and empowered by knowledge, skills, and heightened awareness. Education and evacuation drills are vital to empower people to make life-saving choices.

The third pillar is equity. Disasters can affect all members of society. Therefore, all individuals must be prepared to cope with them. It is a question of justice and an issue of effectiveness. When part of the whole is weak, the entire network becomes more fragile. No one can be left behind. All citizens must be provided with access to basic safety nets. That is why UNESCO emphasizes equal access to education for all children, boys and girls. Half of humankind's collective intelligence and capacity is a resource that cannot be overlooked, especially in times of crisis. Any serious shift toward more resilient societies requires gender equality.

The fourth pillar is to enable individuals faced with trauma to conserve and strengthen their sense of identity and self-esteem by relying on symbolic points of reference. This is a key factor in resilience. It is essential for individuals to feel that they are not merely the plaything of impersonal forces beyond their control, but that they can take their destiny in hand and make choices for the future. Education and reliance on a living culture are tools with considerable and untapped potential for increasing the human capacity for perseverance. UNESCO was one of the first UN agencies to support activities to minimize the effects from the radiation fallout from Chernobyl. The UNESCO Chernobyl Programme (1990) focused on coping with the human dimensions of the catastrophe which were largely underestimated. UNESCO helped set up rehabilitation centers in Belarus, the Russian Federation, and Ukraine to host and counsel people needing social and psychological rehabilitation. The Centers focused on reeducation and information, helping people take care of their own business, diminishing social tension, and reorganizing civil society. They also had a vocation of being experimental educational centers for a new generation of psychologists and social workers.

Lastly, UNESCO works with the UN and other partners to ensure a continuum between emergency relief operations coordinated by the Office for the Coordination of Humanitarian Affairs (OCHA) and sustainable longer-term recovery. We need to shift the "humanitarian versus development" paradigm. To this end, UNESCO works to build bridges between humanitarian and recovery phases and the more long-term development and reconstruction processes. We seek to restore as soon as possible the continuity of a society's educational and cultural fabric, as these are factors of normalization in the event of crisis. We believe this is also vital to "build back better" and to mitigate future damages and loss of life from recurrent and cyclical natural disasters. Following Myanmar's Cyclone Nargis in 2008, UNESCO's Myanmar Education Recovery Programme has worked to support resilience of the education sector through integrating emergency preparedness into the planning and management of the education system. UNESCO also engaged in the delivery of resource packs for township education officers, schools principals, teachers, and an estimated 400,000 students from affected townships. The organization provides technical advice on the construction of hazard-resistant schools and for the protection of cultural heritage. In the aftermath of disasters, UNESCO contributes to the rehabilitation of the educational establishment.

These pillars constitute the focus of UNESCO's work. UNESCO is not a humanitarian agency. Rather, it crafts the conditions to lessen the impact of disasters and build back better. We do not provide the hardware to build stronger societies but the software to make them more resilient.

The implementation of this general principle takes various forms. In the analysis below, I shall present four examples to highlight different aspects of UNESCO's work in the field of tsunami prevention, training for schoolchildren, heritage protection, and the dissemination of humanitarian information.

Knowledge for Prevention: The Example of Tsunami Warning Systems

Large-scale natural disasters rarely affect one country only. The example of tsunami prevention is enlightening in this respect. No single country can develop basin-wide tsunami warning systems. As a catalyst for global scientific cooperation, UNESCO plays a major role in coordinating national warning systems, and in ensuring that national capacities are strengthened in the introduction and monitoring of such mechanisms.

Since 1965, the UNESCO Intergovernmental Oceanographic Commission (IOC) has been responsible for the coordination of the Pacific tsunami warning system. The Indian Ocean tsunami in 2004 gave renewed impetus to the effort to establish early warning systems worldwide, and the IOC was given the mandate to pursue this objective. On October 12, 2011, UNESCO successfully launched the tsunami early warning system in the Indian Ocean, following approximately six years of development work. Similar warning systems are being developed in the Caribbean, North East Atlantic, and Mediterranean and connected seas.

These regional tsunami warning systems are complete end-to-end warning systems, involving advanced technology for data sharing as well as comprehensive learning activities to teach coastal populations about tsunami danger and how to respond to tsunami. UNESCO helps professionals and populations to better anticipate the risks, to assess possible flooding, and to coordinate monitoring.

International scientific cooperation can help in countering such events, whose scope extends beyond frontiers and state capacity, but it cannot replace the authority and initiative of national leaders. We must do much more to strengthen the capacities of local communities so that warnings can reach the people most at risk in good time. With minutes to spare, coastal populations must be able recognize the natural tsunami warning signs and act immediately to save their lives by moving to higher ground.

The example of the tsunami on March 11, 2011, off the coast of Japan illustrates the point. Many coastal tsunami protection structures were destroyed. Indeed, of the 300 kilometers of coastal levees in the To-hoku region, 190 kilometers were fully or partly destroyed. The Fuku-shima nuclear disaster is a direct consequence of this, and we know its implications. In addition, many critical buildings, such as disaster management centers, city-government halls, fire stations, hospitals, and schools were destroyed. This rendered the rapid intervention of the emergency services all the more difficult.

On that day, a major tsunami warning was issued by the Japan Meteorological Agency within three minutes, but the initial warning underestimated the size of the tsunami, and delayed immediate evacuation in some cases.[2] This experience shows the extent to which reducing the impact of a disaster is not merely a question of the system, but also of training and preparation. Early self-evacuation is vital, particularly if a strong earthquake is felt or if the earthquake is weak with slow tremors that continue for a long time. Communities must be capable of assessing the danger for themselves and carrying out immediate evacuations without waiting for official instructions. This is what happened in many schools, such as the Nakano School in Sendai. After the earthquake, the pupils left their classrooms and went to high ground, and so were able to avoid the wave that arrived a few minutes later.

Full-scale simulation exercises are a key element in any disaster-preparedness policy. Such tsunami drills and exercises should include worst-case scenarios, with due consideration for seasonal meteorological conditions and the possibility that primary evacuation routes may be blocked. Underestimated tsunami warnings have an impact on people's reaction, and this is why the content of the national tsunami warnings must be examined from the recipients' point of view.

UNESCO ensures students and teachers are trained in schools across disaster-prone areas. In Latin America, we organized workshops and training sessions in coastal cities in Colombia, Ecuador, Peru, and Chile after the earthquake in 2010. UNESCO also piloted the first full-scale simulation exercise in the Caribbean and neighboring countries on March 23, 2011, with the participation of thirty-three countries and territories, in order to strengthen the defenses of a particularly vulnerable region. Over 300 public and private institutions were associated with the exercise to test communication networks and evacuation procedures.

Experience of tsunamis also brings back memories of past events, as well as traditional knowledge accumulated by communities—in particular indigenous communities—to protect themselves. In some villages on the coast of Japan, stone markers dating back to the late nineteenth century and the tsunami of 1896 indicated the rules to follow in the event of an earthquake. In the village of Aneyoshi, in Iwate province, one of these tsunami stones showed the limit under which residents should not build their houses. Unfortunately, the warnings are not always known or heeded. More often than not, the warnings on the markers have been overlooked, especially in coastal towns which have expanded in the postwar economic boom. In some places, communities installed on the heights have moved down to be closer to their fishing boats.

Indigenous awareness of a tsunami's warning signs saved all but seven members of the population of the Indonesian island of Simeulue off Sumatra in 2004. Traditional houses on the island of Nias in Indonesia are built on intersecting piling and supported by piles of heavy stones in order to resist earthquakes and strong winds. They survived undamaged, while other, more recent dwellings were razed to the ground. In other Indonesian islands, fishermen were used to recognizing the warning signs of a tsunami: the sea suddenly withdrawing and the grasshoppers, usually very noisy at that time of year, falling silent. They immediately sought refuge on elevated ground before the wave arrived. This knowledge should be accessible to all. We should be building modern tsunami stones, and revitalizing this knowledge through land-use planning, using new technologies, and broadcasting warnings through radio and mobile telephones. UNESCO's 2003 Convention for the Safeguarding of the Intangible Cultural Heritage is an instrument that should enable this capital to be shared and enhanced for the benefit of all.

Humanity has unexploited knowledge and capacities. This knowledge and faculty for anticipation are unequally distributed and poorly dispersed or transmitted. They are also fatally difficult to mobilize in emergencies. It is a matter of urgency to restore this knowledge and ensure that all communities can benefit from it. In its role as a clearinghouse for information and international cooperation, UNESCO is playing a major part in this effort. UNESCO seeks to promote the study of natural hazards such as earthquakes, windstorms (cyclones, hurricanes, tornadoes, typhoons), tsunamis, floods, landslides, volcanic eruptions, and droughts, as well as the development of techniques and measures to mitigate risks associated with these types of disasters. UNESCO's international and intergovernmental programs in water sciences, earth sciences, ecological sciences, oceanographic sciences, and engineering sciences mobilize hundreds of scientists and engineers and tens of institutions worldwide, all engaged in disaster studies. Over the past five decades, this network has constituted the backbone behind the contribution of UNESCO to the assessment of hazards, to their distribution in time and space, and to the promotion of techniques for mitigating their effects when they manifest themselves in disasters.

The regional tsunami information centers are a core component of UNESCO's strategy to train local populations. These centers are repositories of awareness and outreach materials, they coordinate training, and they provide technical advice. UNESCO is working to develop these centers and to enhance States' ability to develop preparedness and awareness. In Africa, operational experience for drought forecasting remains very limited at the regional and national level. UNESCO has developed a comprehensive set of integrated water-resources management guidelines at river-basin level, which includes special volumes for managing floods and drought. It must be possible for strong institutions at the local, national, and international levels to manage this knowledge and to build a "culture of safety." The foundations for this culture are laid at school.

Resilience Starts in Schools

Disasters show that there is no barrier that cannot be overcome, no embankment or protection that cannot be damaged. The hardiest protection is that which is built in the minds of men and women, and this starts with education. Education provides sustainability to all disaster risk reduction initiatives. It can help build the foundations for more resilient societies that are able to respond and adapt to the pressures of change. Education is also an extremely powerful "weapon of mass prevention." In March 2011, at the launch of UNESCO's *Education for All Global Monitoring Report*, the Right Honourable Michaëlle Jean, UNESCO Special Envoy for Haiti, remarked that "education is a precious commodity that no earthquake in the world can ever remove from the mind of a child who has been to school."[3]

It is important to identify three aspects of the role of education in disaster management. First, as a fundamental right of every human being, basic education is indispensable for accessing information and being able to interpret it, in normal times as well as in times of crisis. Quality education for all is a formidable shock absorber in a crisis and a powerful stabilizer of society. Illiteracy is a cause of vulnerability and dependency in individuals. Being unable to read and write considerably limits people's capacities to make choices and to take control of their lives—whether through reading information signs, learning how to guard against diseases such as HIV/AIDS, or informing oneself on all aspects of everyday life. This vulnerability can be fatal in extreme situations. General basic education is an essential investment for anticipating crises.

A second aspect concerns education about risks as such. This means raising the awareness of individuals and training them from a very young age, for instance, in first aid in the event of disaster. A central element of this strategy consists of linking together education in risk reduction and education in sustainable development. As the lead agency for the United Nations Decade of Education for Sustainable Development, UNESCO makes every effort to ensure that this link is explicit in school curricula and activities. It is essential to build a culture of safety and resilience at all levels, in line with the priorities of the Hyogo Framework for Action (2005–15) adopted by 168 countries in 2005. The Framework explicitly refers to the important role of education.

Schoolchildren and students should understand the fundamental link between the protection of the environment and the prevention of natural hazards. It is important for learners to understand what to do when a disaster occurs and how to design their communities in a way that make them more resilient against disasters—for instance, with regard to how their houses are built. Especially in cases when the reasons for hazards are man-made or exacerbated by humans, learners must understand these causes and be empowered to do something against them. In simple terms, learners must know how to adapt in practical terms to rising sea levels and they should be empowered to do something against climate change.

Education can support the mitigation and prevention of the human causes of disasters on a long-term basis. The UNESCO Climate Change Education for Sustainable Development program explicitly includes disaster risk reduction in its activities and tools. Our aim is to support States to strengthen their educational responses to mitigate and adapt to climate change, including through education for disaster preparedness. We have developed, for instance, a teacher-education course to strengthen the capacities of education policymakers to integrate climate change and disaster risk reduction into polices and curricula as well as teacher-training institutions. The focus has fallen especially on Africa and Small Island Developing States (SIDS).

The Sandwatch program provides insight to UNESCO's work. This is a volunteer network of schools, youth groups, and nongovernmental and community-based organizations that was initiated in the Caribbean in 1999. It has become global since then, with a focus on SIDS. From the Cook Islands in the Pacific and the Seychelles in the Indian Ocean to the Bahamas in the Caribbean, Sandwatch seeks to modify the lifestyles and habits of children, youth, and adults by developing awareness of the fragile nature of the marine and coastal environment.

We believe this is crucial, because half of the world's population lives on the coast. Fourteen of the world's seventeen mega-cities (with at least 10 million inhabitants) are situated less than 200 kilometers from a sea. The world's coastal-area population is set to double by 2025. Urbanization is weakening vital ecosystems like coral reefs and mangroves that provide natural protection against tsunamis. Some 70 percent of beaches in the world today suffer from rapid erosion—because of human activities and short-term development requirements. Protection of these marine and coastal ecosystems is a shared responsibility. Mismanagement of natural resources, the leveling of slopes, and deforestation also increase the impact of flooding, which then inundates large areas causing considerable damage on land leveled by human activity. Developing a culture of safety must be taken forward in the widest sense—looking beyond urban planning toward a global understanding of the environment. In this respect, UNESCO's broad mandate provides a real comparative advantage in emergency education.

UNESCO works to include disaster risk reduction into school curricula within an "education for sustainable development" framework. With the United Nations Children's Fund (UNICEF), we have undertaken a global mapping of the integration of disaster risk reduction into curricula that captures key national experiences and good practices in twenty-nine countries. Disaster risk reduction is still integrated into only a narrow band of subjects, typically the physical and natural sciences. This is why together with UNICEF and with funding from the government of Japan, UNESCO is developing an international technical guidance instrument for education planners and curriculum specialists. This will provide a rationale for including disaster risk reduction into curricula and relevant knowledge to be acquired by learners at different levels of education. It will guide those with responsibility for curricula on teaching and learning methods to empower and motivate learners and to support the development of a comprehensive culture of disaster resilience. UNESCO's *Education for Sustainable Development Lens: A Policy and Practice Review Tool* helps policymakers, education officials, and curriculum specialists to reorient education toward sustainable development. It can also be used to integrate disaster risk reduction in national education plans and specific curricula.

A third aspect is the challenge of integrating the educational dimension into the very early stages of the emergency response to disasters. Emergency education can have a lifesaving impact. It must be a central part of any core emergency humanitarian response, enabling children and the community to regain a sense of normalcy following the disaster. UNESCO's work on temporary schools in Peru following the earthquake in 2007 served as a basis for early recovery and development.[4] Much more must be done here. Although UNESCO's educational programs increasingly integrate humanitarian operations coordinated by OCHA, education still remains a tiny fraction of humanitarian investment— representing just 2 percent of humanitarian aid.[5] Education is the poor cousin of a humanitarian aid system that is underfunded, unpredictable, and governed by short-termism. The potential of education to save lives is still underplayed in the entire humanitarian cycle—this must change.

Culture on the Front Line

In recent years, disasters have had a heavy impact on UNESCO World Heritage sites, resulting in the loss of lives and causing vast damage.[6] In 2007, Cyclone Sidr in the Sundarbans (Bangladesh) led to the destruction of forest and mangroves, the drowning of fishermen and wildlife, and saltwater intrusion. In September 2011, northern Luzon (Philippines) was severely affected by Typhoon Pedring, whose trajectory passed across the Ifugao province and caused major mud and landslides within the area of the World Heritage property of the Rice Terraces in the Philippine Cordilleras. The vulnerability of these sites has become a major concern because of the role that heritage plays for the confidence and dignity of people throughout the world. Concerns also arise because of culture's crucial contribution to sustainable development, especially at times of diminishing resources.

UNESCO has a long experience in building the capacities of States and site managers to anticipate disaster risks and to protect themselves against destructive consequences. In response to a call from the Pakistani government, UNESCO launched in 1974 an international campaign to safeguard and consolidate the archaeological ruins at Moenjodaro, situated in the province of Sindh. For over twenty years, UNESCO guided the construction of five enormous dams on the Indus floodplain in order to protect the site from flooding. This international campaign was completed in 1997 and enabled local know-how to emerge for the protection of the site and the establishment of a laboratory for conservation and monitoring. The operation raised the awareness of 150 million people about Moenjodaro and the civilization of the Indus. It is largely thanks to this support and the training of local people that the site was saved from the terrible floods of the summer of 2010. The protection of heritage sites is a process without an end. Even efforts to protect Moenjodaro were not able to totally safeguard the site from the flooding that hit the valley in 2011.

In the face of these challenges, the number of World Heritage properties that have developed a proper disaster risk management plan is surprisingly low. This situation is especially worrying, as experience shows that heritage sites can help to reduce the impact of disasters when they are well managed. This is true not only for natural heritage resources that guarantee the proper functioning of ecosystems—the maintaining of embankments, forests, and landforms that play a role as natural shock absorbers in the event of flooding—but also for cultural heritage properties that, as a result of traditional knowledge accumulated over centuries of adaptation to environmental conditions, have proved resilient to disasters while providing shelter and psychological support to affected communities.

In 2007, the World Heritage Committee adopted a Strategy for Reducing Disaster Risks and has developed a series of programmatic and capacity-building tools to assist in its implementation and provide methodology for assessing and reducing risks.[7] The operations to clean the Borobudur Temple Compounds in Indonesia, which were covered with corrosive ash following the eruption of Mount Merapi in November 2010, are particularly revealing in this regard.

The Borobudur Temple Compounds, built in Central Java around 800 A.D., are considered one of the greatest religious monuments on earth. It is the most visited tourist attraction in Indonesia and a pilgrimage site for Buddhists from all over the world. In the case of Borobudur, UNESCO sought to implement the most comprehensive safeguarding plan possible. More than just a rescue campaign, the project has helped mobilize the potential of culture as a motor for development and engagement for the entire local community.[8] It is an illustration of the "build back better" concept.

From January 2011 until December 2011, the UNESCO office in Jakarta—in collaboration with the Ministry of Culture and Tourism and local nongovernmental organizations (NGOs)—deployed some 570 workers from the local community to clear ash from the monument. The local community members—who were coordinated by local NGOs—worked five days a week to clear the ash. In December 2011, after close to a year of cleaning, these operations were completed successfully and the temple was officially reopened to the public.

In addition to the clean-up operations and building the science capacities of local experts and curators, UNESCO worked to turn the disaster into an opportunity for the local craft and tourist sectors. With the Ministry of Culture and Tourism, UNESCO increased training activities in local crafts as part of a global strategy to empower the local communities. This has meant activities for livelihood and income generation through cultural industries, such as cultural tourism management programs, craft-based training programs in traditional activities (textile weaving, bamboo/cane/banana leaf weaving), wood craft, manufacture of religious artifacts, stone carving, and other related handicrafts. In the course of the safeguarding operation, 45 cubic meters of ash from the Borobudur temple were collected along with an abundance of lava stone from the volcano's eruption. In a surprising and productive turnaround, all of this could be used for the production of unique, regional crafts.

The participants also learned skills that they can pass on to the local communities. This included sessions on design and how to create attractive products—helping them create lucrative small businesses which would improve local livelihoods. Other training activities have been added in the field of tourism, hospitality, and gastronomy.

On the whole, this project is one of the most successful examples of an all-around response to an event of this type, in which the involvement of local communities resulted in the overhaul of an entire sector of activities. It shows how the implementation of UNESCO's cultural conventions has also been a successful development strategy. Culture is not a luxury. It is a valuable investment in times of diminishing resources, one that promotes a capital that local populations are best equipped to maintain and enhance over the long term.

UNESCO is campaigning to change the perception of culture's role in disaster response. The cultural dimension must be integrated from the first stages of emergency operations. The organization is working with other UN agencies (including the United Nations Development Programme and World Bank) and the European Union to integrate a cultural component within the Post-Disaster Needs Assessment process.

Information Saves Lives

As other chapters of this publication demonstrate, reliable and accurate sources of information in local languages can support national and international efforts to save lives, livelihoods, and resources. UNESCO also plays a role here, as the lead specialized agency for communication and information. There can be no real disaster risk reduction or preparation without massive assistance from the media, nor without the proactive use of social media. In this respect, SMS chains in disasters are perhaps the best and most obvious example. Following a disaster, communication and information allow victims to quickly find out about what happened and where to go for help.

Following the earthquake in Haiti, for instance, UNESCO organized training for Haitian journalists on disaster risk mitigation with l'Association des journalistes haïtiens and in cooperation with the Haitian civil protection department. This training involved 380 journalists in nine departments of the country. Such training is important to provide practical exercises for media professionals on how to communicate information in local languages following a disaster, applying humanitarian information made available from the UN Country Team as well as other reliable sources. In Haiti and elsewhere, UNESCO makes great use of its "radio-in-a-box." This is a mobile transmitter that can be carried to different locations in the event of natural disasters. Even if local radio stations are unable to transmit in a city, the "radio-in-a-box" can disseminate emergency humanitarian messages to affected populations.

Working for the Long Term

For the last 10,000 years, the planet's environment has been unusually stable. This period of stability—known to geologists as the Holocene—has come to an end, and since the Industrial Revolution, a new era has emerged, the Anthropocene, in which human actions are the main driver of global change.[9] Our planet is under unprecedented stress.

How can we provide greater stability and predictability in an increasingly unpredictable world? No agency or country can react alone. This requires collective work over the long term, underpinned by a firm commitment to forge ahead. The difficulty is also that a disaster that is avoided has a lower profile than one that is not.

We must strengthen our collective capacity to evolve in a context of uncertainty and increased risk. Above all, we must identify the enablers that are most likely to consolidate the resilience of people facing the increase of extreme events. We must also rethink the risk anticipation and information-sharing models that are vital for better understanding and managing uncertainties. As stated in the report of the UN Secretary-General's High-level Panel on Global Sustainability, we must define what scientists refer to as "planetary boundaries," "environmental thresholds," and "tipping points."[10]

Risk is no longer an external threat, but a building block of society. This new "risk society" urges us to build a corresponding "culture of safety and resilience." Vulnerability reduction is an overriding objective guiding UNESCO's work. Disaster risk reduction is a horizontal theme cutting across all of our areas of competence. UNESCO works for an integrated approach to building disaster resilient communities. We encourage stronger linkages of disaster risk reduction elements across the fields of sustainable development. Synergies save lives—this integrated approach is the basis for a more effective disaster risk management.

Toward a Culture of Safety and Resilience

This concept of humanitarian effectiveness, which seeks to build people's capacities to respond to crises themselves, fits with a vision of human development that seeks to widen the choices available to individuals and their ability to react in real situations. A development strategy without the active participation of the target populations is doomed to failure. The same rule applies to efforts to manage disasters without the full, agreed, and controlled involvement of those concerned.

The challenge is to identify what drives this participation and involvement. In its report submitted to UNESCO in 1995, the World Commission on Culture and Development highlighted the need to take into account the cultural dimension of societies, to elicit support from the people, and to formulate development policies that may be permanently established.[11] Culture is a compass that individuals use to navigate in the real world and to shape it in the ways they wish. It is also a strategic enabler that encourages the participation of individuals and helps them to adapt to events beyond their control. While the indivisibility of culture and sustainable development is recognized, a similar movement must take place in the field of crisis management. This must also include the intangible resources that are transmitted by school, through heritage, and in knowledge-sharing in ways that strengthen the resilience of societies. All of these must be firmly integrated into crisis management efforts. This can also lay the foundation for more effective development policies. By definition, *human* development and *sustainable* development must be *resilient*.

Building a culture of resilience is a core part of UNESCO's pursuit of a wider culture of peace. In the twenty-first century, this must include promoting mutual understanding between peoples and their participation in sustainable development, along with the ability to cope with disasters. There can be no lasting peace when societies remain at the mercy of natural hazards. The resulting population movements, struggles for access to water, and conflicts over the control of critical resources are all risks to global stability. Faced with these risks, human ingenuity is our greatest asset. This humanist vision inspired the creation of UNESCO in 1945. At a time of rapid change, this vision has never been so relevant.

Education and Disaster Management

KEVIN M. CAHILL, M.D., AND
ALEXANDER VAN TULLEKEN, M.D.

Growth and Expertise

Total emergency relief aid spending has increased significantly in the last forty odd years. In 1970 total emergency aid spending was less than $1 billion per year. This figure began to rise sharply in the 1990s, and by 2010 annual spending was over $20 billion per year.[1] The end of the Cold War, the subsequent proliferations of civil wars, and their consequent displacement crises in the 1990s certainly suggest that this increase in spending was driven in part by a concomitant increase in need. A decade into the twenty-first century we are able to observe the "humanitarian international"[2]—the vast complex of international organizations endeavoring to deliver humanitarian assistance—as a globally powerful entity, with capabilities and ambitions far beyond what existed in the early 1970s.

But it is legitimate to ask if the vast expansion in spending represents phenomena beyond simple moral progress in foreign policy to address suffering. We are also compelled to ask what changes in practice and in attitude can be observed in the individuals and organizations that make up the "humanitarian international" in the context of such rapid growth. This book poses an essential and timely question: How can we do *More with Less*? It is, however, important to remember that the question presented to many humanitarian organizations through the last four decades has been: How can we do *more* with *more*?

The rapid expansion of humanitarian aid has been accompanied by extensive commentary on the successes and failures of vast aid operations; on the delivery of goods and services;[3] on the need for minimum standards; and on the need for training and qualifications for aid workers. Professionalization and accountability have, time and again, been suggested as panaceas for the persistent, significant flaws in humanitarian responses to disasters and emergencies.[4] Concerned individuals, departments, and institutions dedicated to promoting professionalization and accountability are clearly emerging.

A New Discipline

It is difficult to describe the moment at which a new profession is recognized. Historically professions have emerged through a mixture of public and private interests, associations between practitioners and academics, state institutions and private ones. These processes are messy, time–consuming, and essential. At Fordham University's Institute of International Humanitarian Affairs (IIHA), our faculty has been engaged in these processes for decades, attempting to shape humanitarian practice while avoiding the pitfalls of creating a system that benefits the professionals more than those it claims to serve.[5]

In the context of increasing demand for qualifications and professional structures, the current reduction in available funding for nongovernmental organizations (NGOs) will have significant effects: donors wish to see improved outcomes, to find ways of justifying spending and discriminating between agencies. NGOs need to find ways of distinguishing themselves and their programs in a competitive environment of increased emphasis on accountability, cost-effectiveness, and the qualifications of staff. Individual aid workers also need to find ways of distinguishing themselves from their colleagues in an increasingly crowded job market. These factors all contribute to the increasing demand for training, qualifications, and moves toward professionalization.

The most indispensable resource in disaster preparedness and response is trained personnel. At the local level disaster preparations must be instilled in the community psyche: children in tornado-prone areas drilled in where to seek safe shelter; in flood-prone areas where and when to seek higher ground. At the regional and national level training of civil servants should be an essential part of public protection. Courses in disaster management are usually required as an ongoing part of all careers that hold potential responsibility for vulnerable populations. Mayors, school teachers, hospital administrators, urban planners, and first responders such as police, fire brigade, ambulance, and search and rescue teams have mandatory programs to keep them abreast of new techniques, changes in geography and climate, and levels of risk. At the international level the United Nations (UN) promotes training and risk reduction awareness as among its top priorities.

The Role of the University

The academy, particularly in the case of a university with a multidisciplinary faculty, has an indispensable influence. It has played an essential role in shaping modern humanitarian assistance, a discipline broad enough, like medicine, to incorporate the many different specialties that are needed to provide comprehensive care in crises.

Only the university can provide the legitimacy and credibility needed in a new world where globalization and international regulations guide all our actions, including the provision of disaster relief.[6] Only a university, empowered by government departments of education, can confer degrees and diplomas. This is absolutely critical for a discipline such as humanitarian assistance, where multiple skills, mandates, and qualifications must be brought under the same umbrella. By its very nature, experts in humanitarian work must be recognized as such by many nations, since those afflicted by war and disaster flee across borders seeking safe havens in neighboring lands.

Humanitarian assistance is a noble undertaking. At an individual level it is as old as mankind, with tales of generosity and compassion being part of the myths, legends, and foundations of every society. As a formal discipline, however, the organized response to the chaos and suffering that is inevitably a part of armed conflicts, or extraordinary natural disasters, has slowly, very slowly, evolved. Codes of conduct were used by ancient Greek city-states in warfare, but it was several thousand years before they were widely accepted as part of international law.

In modern times there has been a growing realization that both innocent victims and injured combatants deserve protection. Henry Dunant's attempt to establish neutral, "universal" space for humanitarian aid in 1859 in the midst of the Battle of Solferino is often cited as the beginning of what we now accept as international humanitarian law. The Geneva Conventions were later established to codify humankind's rules for the treatment of civilians and the injured, as well as for the behavior of combatants. The implementation of the Conventions has sadly been a tale of constant exceptions and shameful interpretations.

In the Spanish Civil War, for example, both sides violated the most basic rules of civilized behavior, denying aid and food to the wounded, and indiscriminately executing women and children. World War II's appalling record of genocide, with barely a response from humanitarian organizations, has continued in the numerous small wars that have scarred the landscapes of Africa, Asia, and Latin America in the last half of the twentieth century. One has only to think back to the horrors of, and bitter struggles in, Rwanda, Sudan, Somalia, the Congo, Sri Lanka, the Balkans, or Nicaragua to recall tens of millions internally displaced persons and refugees who had lost all, fleeing aimlessly without adequate help.

At the close of the Cold War humanitarian assistance entered an era of enormous complexity, and it was ill prepared for the challenges that aid agencies faced. There were no universally accepted standards for providing care in such dire situations. There were few comprehensive training programs; in fact there was not even a common vocabulary for guiding humanitarian workers. Academia was not seen as part of the solution, and its absence added to the problems.

Humanitarian assistance, practiced in the midst of conflicts and disasters, is not a field for amateurs. Good intentions are a common, but tragically inadequate, substitute for well-planned, efficiently coordinated and carefully implemented operations that, like a good sentence, must have a beginning, middle, and an end. Compassion and charity are only elements in humanitarian assistance programs; alone they are self-indulgent emotions that, for a short time, may satisfy the donor but will always fail to help victims in desperate straits. What was desperately needed was the creation of a new discipline, one that could embrace the many areas of expertise required to provide an overall response. This is where the university and academia had to enter the picture.

It is primarily in the university, the academy, where knowledge is analyzed and defined, where good—and bad—practices are studied, where the lessons of the past are distilled in a continuing search for wisdom and understanding. Humanitarian assistance is an ideal—if long neglected—area for academic interest. It presents a multidisciplinary challenge, drawing on, among others, the fields of public health and medicine, law and politics, logistics and security, technology and anthropology, indeed all the social, physical, moral, economic, and philosophic sciences.

The complex causes of, and difficult solutions to, humanitarian crises require an arena for the free, unfettered exchange of ideas, where the development of innovative approaches is encouraged to overcome the failed status quo. That is the essential environment of a good university. The university should be—and usually is—the last bastion where open discussions, and respect for differing ideas, prevail. It is society's ultimate refuge from bias and prejudice, and these are among the most significant causative factors in humanitarian crises.

Universities are founded to preserve the best in our traditions, to use the collection of data and the wisdom that flows from study to elevate the physical, mental, and spiritual lives of all. It is patently obvious that universities—to fulfill their most basic mission—must devote their diverse skills and talents to assist those unfortunate segments of humankind caught in the maelstrom of wars or made homeless—and often helpless—by natural disasters.

A lasting respect between those in need and those who have the privilege to give can occur, and this is one of the foundations on which we can build bridges to peace.[7] Every university must be part of the everyday struggles of mankind. There are no ivory towers that should—or can—isolate intellectuals from the masses. Ideally, the ultimate calling of the university should be to help those most in need, to apply wisdom in order to right wrongs and relieve suffering.

Society has entrusted universities with establishing rigorous standards to assure good practices. In every country, for example, one must pass an academic exam to practice as a doctor or a lawyer; in fact, in the United States one must qualify, by academic testing, to be a plumber or a hairdresser. Yet until recently there have been no standards required to become a humanitarian worker. One only had to have—or contend one had—a big heart, lots of compassion. Too often "humanitarian workers" went to crisis situations to fulfill their own needs, to gratify their own dreams, to satisfy a distorted sense of redemption in a place of chaos. Many had no training, few skills, and even fewer inner resources to sustain them. These deluded volunteers complicated relief efforts, often causing more harm than good. An inordinate amount of time was spent helping to extricate them from refugee camps, draining vital energies that should have been devoted to the real victims of disasters.

Early in the 1990s, a brief survey by the IIHA of training requirements revealed that, even within the UN system, there were widely varying courses and no record of qualifications. International NGOs often functioned with haphazard training and no understanding of the specific roles of other aid agencies or, for that matter, of the people they were there to assist. They spent precious time in competition with local aid groups and among themselves.

Such experiences led humanitarian workers to the university to establish consistent requirements for appropriate training for all who presumed to enter turbulent zones of disaster and share in the inordinately satisfying task of dispensing critical assistance. Over the past few decades there has been a slow but steady progress in developing formal university courses in humanitarian action, with some academic centers now offering undergraduate programs as well as graduate-level degrees in this discipline.

The Fordham Experience

Fordham University in New York established the IIHA in the mid-1990s. It has, as of 2012, trained over 1,800 graduates in all aspects of humanitarian response. The average age of our candidates is mid- to late thirties: they are mostly experienced field practitioners who have demonstrated a longer commitment than is ordinarily seen in the high turnover of staff of many agencies. Most importantly they come from over 133 nations.

The IIHA aims to create a community of practice through organized training courses that emphasizes the core mission of humanitarian aid: a people-centered response to suffering, according to need, motivated by humanity. Our courses are designed to be accessible to aid workers from the Global South, and particularly from crisis-affected populations. We have held courses on five continents in over twenty countries. By offering training in locations such as Sudan, Kenya, Malaysia, Myanmar, and Nicaragua we reduce travel costs, bring training closer to the field, and alleviate the visa problems faced by many students from the Global South when seeking education in North America or Europe. Almost 25 percent of our student body is comprised of local staff whose training is heavily supported by scholarships.

Local staff comprises the vast bulk of aid workers, and yet this group has the least access to high-quality training. In an era when the humanitarian space is threatened and competition for funds is intense, aid agencies often seem to be more accountable to donors rather than affected populations. When integrated mission and political instrumentalization are real challenges to humanitarian principles, the inclusion of affected populations in meaningful and substantive participation in the strategies and priorities of the response, as well as the response itself, must be an essential consideration in any training program. Because the modular design of the Fordham Master's training program does not require long periods away from full-time work, local candidates are able return to the field rapidly to implement their training.

The IDHA

The IIHA, in conjunction with partners at the City University of New York, University of Geneva, University of Liverpool, the Liverpool School of Tropical Medicine, the Royal College of Surgeons in Ireland,

and the UN System Staff College, has offered qualifications in humanitarian assistance for the past fifteen years. Our premier course, the International Diploma in Humanitarian Assistance (IDHA),[8] was developed to respond to the lack of skills and training that was so detrimental to many humanitarian responses in the last decades of the twentieth century. The IDHA qualification has now been incorporated into a Master's degree in International Humanitarian Assistance (MIHA) and has kept pace with the rapid change of tools and technologies available to relief workers.

The IDHA is a month-long residential course that was designed to simulate the hard realities of fieldwork in a humanitarian crisis. Students live in dormitory accommodation, with the forced intimacy of shared meals, working up to fourteen hours each day and five and a half days a week for a full month. They participate in seminars and meetings, exercises, and debates, absorbing and discussing the views of expert faculty and exchanging ideas based on their own experiences. All faculty have extensive practical experience in natural and man-made disasters.

Candidates are graded according to strict academic standards; a significant portion of their total grade is based on their work as a member of a "syndicate" of five to seven members who work throughout the month as a coordinated team. This approach is based on the absolute necessity for close cooperation in crisis situations. Each IDHA program has between thirty-five and forty-five candidates, a staff of five or six tutors, and guest lecturers as available. Because of the wonder of the internet, IDHA graduates tend to stay in close contact after graduation, and often discover each other in refugee camps years after their course. As of 2012, we have held thirty-nine IDHA programs, thrice annually: in New York City, in Geneva, Switzerland, and a third program somewhere in Africa, Latin America, or Asia.

The MIHA

The MIHA program is available to IDHA graduates who wish to pursue a more advanced academic degree. It is made up of four modules: the

IDHA; the International Diploma in Operational Humanitarian Assistance; the International Diploma in the Management of Humanitarian Action; and the International Diploma in Humanitarian Leadership. This modular structure makes the degree flexible enough to fit into humanitarians' professional schedules. Courses are offered in one-, two-, and four-week intensive sessions in locations around the world including Spain, Switzerland, Kenya, India, Turkey, Egypt, Ireland, Indonesia, Dublin, Kuala Lumpur, New York, and South Africa.

Elective courses within the modules include, among others, humanitarian logistics; ethics of humanitarian assistance; management and leadership; mental health in complex emergencies; humanitarian negotiations; civil-military cooperation; human rights and humanitarian law; forced migration; and the role of the media in disasters. These courses emphasize technical skills and service delivery which are essential in an environment where technologies and tools change rapidly, where donors and agency headquarters demand ever higher standards and more sophisticated metrics for monitoring and evaluation.

In addition to the practical, field-oriented teachers, the training programs also draw on a wide range of Fordham faculty from the Graduate School of Arts and Sciences, the School of Law, School of Business, and the School of Social Service. These teachers bring to bear on humanitarian endeavors academic skills of critical analysis and theoretical work. Leaders in the humanitarian field should be able to understand, for example, the demographics of an affected population, their needs in terms of water and sanitation, and the ways in which a program meeting these needs might be planned, managed, funded, and evaluated. But aid workers, even with the training and expertise needed for such technical projects, are at risk of losing sight of the significance and complexity of the problems they address.

Therefore, they must also be trained to understand the nature of the relationship between a beleaguered population and its government, the subtle mechanisms by which humanitarianism can be instrumentalized for political purposes, and the ways in which donors, the media, their own agencies, and host governments can use the metrics generated by a program to shape a wide variety of narratives serving a similarly wide variety of purposes. An aid worker, with even the highest level of technical skills, can inadvertently become an agent of abusive governments' attempts to manipulate and control their populations. Situating humanitarian training within the university allows us to draw on critical thinking of the academy in ways that helps candidates comprehend a very complex world, and then, hopefully, act appropriately.

Our candidates, for example, would study not only the ways in which food might be delivered to a starving population, and the particular kinds of food that might be most useful and acceptable, but also what it means to bear witness to starvation in the language of biostatistics. They analyze what is lost and what is gained in the ways in which we choose to represent a starving population. Are they utterly helpless, or do they represent a group of people whose main problem is lack of food complicated by a lack of political access?

Our Master's graduates should be able to analyze the complex realities of poverty, suffering, and security, to see the concealed forces that shape humanitarian assistance and the vested interests in humanitarian responses. They should be able to discuss the relationship between the citizen and the state, and the nature of power in ways that will inform their understanding of the government structures that emerge, or are concealed, within a billion-dollar, state-sponsored humanitarian industry.

The Undergraduate Program

The IIHA also offers an academic program aimed at undergraduate students, the International Humanitarian Affairs (IHA) Minor. This unique six-course interdisciplinary program provides students with insights into the complex issues central to contemporary humanitarian affairs, seen through the academic lenses of political science, international studies, history, sociology, philosophy, and theology. Students examine the global impact of natural and man-made disasters, disease, poverty, conflict, human rights violations, international law, as well as government and intergovernmental policies on international human communities.

Two of the most popular courses included in the IHA Minor are the Foreign Service Program and the International Humanitarian Affairs Internship Seminar. The Foreign Service Program introduces students in their final year of undergraduate study to the experience of international humanitarian aid work through a preparatory semester followed by an organized field study in a region affected by natural or human-made disaster. The course and travel component equip students with firsthand experience and knowledge of the social, economic, political, and environmental issues of the region. As the capstone course, the IHA Internship Seminar gives students an opportunity to gain practical experience in the field as an intern for an international humanitarian organization prior to graduation. These two courses equip students with skills only taught through real-life experience.

Additionally, undergraduates studying humanitarian affairs at Fordham can also participate in a biannual national conference with students from the other twenty-eight Jesuit universities in the United States through the Jesuit Universities Humanitarian Action Network,[9] of which Fordham is a founding partner.

Conclusion

The university has become an essential partner in international humanitarian assistance. Untrained workers are now rarely accepted, even as volunteers, by major NGOs and reputable international organizations. An academic diploma in humanitarian assistance has become a sine qua non as relief workers increasingly move from the UN and national relief organizations to the private sector, and back. The imprimatur offered by a highly respected, university-legitimized, diploma, based on practical experience, is now appreciated around the world.

Senior humanitarian workers also now take advantage of the opportunity to periodically retreat to an academic setting where the multidisciplinary nature of humanitarian assistance is reviewed, and updated analyses of good—and bad—practices are considered. Those specializing in one aspect of relief work have the opportunity to share with, and learn from, those who may see the same crisis from utterly different perspectives.

Preserving humanitarian space is imperative. This presents a formidable challenge, and only the education of a committed cadre of trained professionals will be able to preserve the traditions of neutrality, impartiality, and independence that make international humanitarian work a noble undertaking.

Disaster management is an evolving discipline and imaginative, creative ideas can often be found by moving beyond the traditional confines of our profession. While conceiving this book, colleagues from the business world were consulted, and they offered ideas that caused me to seek the input of those who study and direct big business.

One might not immediately relate tourism and disasters, but the sheer scope of travel offers potential in both preparedness, and in response. Three distinguished entrepreneurs then offer their own unique insights and experiences, and end this text on an optimistic note. Somehow we can emerge as a better world if everyone, in every profession, is welcomed to participate in disaster preparedness and response.

Capitalizing on Travel and Tourism in Preparing for Trouble

RICHARD GORDON

In January 2005, ironically only days after the Indian Ocean tsunami had claimed 225,000 lives and displaced 1.2 million others, representatives from 168 governments met in Hyogo, Japan, to discuss and then sign a historic framework. The framework, entitled the Hyogo Framework for Action (HFA), seeks to encourage nations to embed the vital issue of disaster risk reduction and preparedness into the everyday processes of national and local governance. It has at its heart the aim of reducing every nation's vulnerability to disasters and, in the event that major hazards strike, the ability to respond in such a way as to minimize loss of life, property, and damage to the environment.[1]

The HFA is not legally binding and thus its implementation across the 168 participating nations has inevitably met with mixed results. Many governments have demonstrated a high dependence upon external leadership, particularly in the form of funding, to attract them to the task of developing integrated risk reduction strategies within their institutions.

The United Nations International Strategy for Disaster Reduction (UNISDR) has provided much of this leadership and funding, helping to establish local committees, national secretariats, regional bodies, and global forums.[2] The governments of numerous developed countries have augmented the work of UNISDR. Additional programs have been designed and funded to assist in the recruitment and training of staff to carry out the essential functions of emergency management, to meet the targets set by the HFA, and to regularly report back on their progress.

As a direct result of this work, national disaster management platforms have been successfully established in many countries. Nevertheless, a midterm literature review[3] commissioned by UNISDR reported in 2011 that ongoing international funding and leadership appeared to remain a vital precondition for further progress in implementing the HFA. It is such funding which is at risk during harsh economic climates and which demands the question as to whether more can be achieved with less.

In 2007 the UNISDR published a set of guidelines entitled *Words into Action*,[4] which sought to give participating governments suggested strategies to adopt in implementing the HFA. These included the identification of, and engagement with, all relevant institutions, mechanisms, and capacities to ensure that every possible activity of national life contributed to the overall task of disaster management. Included within the guidelines was a suggested list of stakeholders that was considered important to the development of any national disaster risk reduction and response framework.[5] Interestingly, although aspects of travel were referred to in the guidelines, travel and tourism as an industry was not specifically mentioned. While no list can be exhaustive, it is argued in this chapter that travel and tourism is a key contributor to the tasks of risk reduction, disaster response, and recovery, and should thus be incorporated as a way of achieving *More with Less*.

What Is Travel and Tourism and Why Is It important?

The United Nations World Tourism Organization (UNWTO) defines tourism as "the activities of persons traveling to and staying in places outside their usual environment for not more than one consecutive year for leisure, business and other purposes."[6] However, since tourists, including the business and "MICE" sector (Meetings, Incentives, Conventions and Exhibitions) demand an infrastructure of hotels, attractions, transportation, and amenities, Macintosh and Goeldner (1986) offer a more detailed industry description. They define tourism as "a collection of activities, services and industries that delivers a travel experience including transportation, accommodations, eating and drinking establishments, retail shops, entertainment businesses, activity facilities and other hospitality services provided for individuals or groups traveling away from home."[7] This definition provides a much fuller description of what is referred to in this chapter as the "travel and tourism industry" and helps to explain the relevance of the sector to the tasks of emergency planning and response.

The travel and tourism industry provides employment, investment and, in some cases, valuable foreign exchange. Today, the industry is a multisector global activity that is present in almost every country on the planet. In financial terms, it accounts for 5 percent of world gross domestic product (GDP) ($3.5 trillion) and 6 percent of total exports (receipts) amounting to $1 trillion including transportation.[8] Its growth over the last forty years has created the fourth-largest export category worldwide after fuels, chemicals, and automotive products.[9]

In 2011, despite challenges in the global economy, political unrest in the Middle East and North Africa, and ongoing natural disasters in many parts of the world, international tourist arrivals grew by 4.4 percent to 980 million.[10] Approximately 51 percent of these tourists travel for leisure, recreation, and holidays; 15 percent travel for business purposes, and the remainder are both visiting friends and family or are traveling to a destination for religious, health, or other reasons.[11]

Clearly, the resilience of such an industry to external events such as disasters is of vital relevance to any economic recovery. It is for this reason that the overriding aim of ministries of tourism, and their related agencies, remains the ongoing marketing of tourism destinations. Even in the midst of a major crisis, tourism ministries will continue to encourage new and old visitors to travel to their country with a thousand variations on the theme "open for business as usual."

Yet all this ignores a vital truth. Travel and tourism is not just a sector of economic activity to be regenerated in the event of a disaster. Neither is it simply another set of victims to be managed by the emergency services. Travel and tourism is, by its very nature, a crucial partner in the development and conduct of any wider strategy for disaster management.

Consider the following similarities: both travel and tourism and emergency managers plan and operate at an international, national, regional, and local level. In both cases their activities affect, and indeed depend upon, the safety of local communities. They are faced with situations, both foreseen and unforeseen, that have, by definition, overwhelmed their capacity using everyday resources. As a result they both require their operations and logistics to be integrated in as efficient a way as possible across communities at the regional, national, and even international levels. In times of emergency they both depend heavily upon the same limited resources including hospitals, medical teams, transportation, evacuation centers, temporary shelters, food and water distribution points, and both contribute to, and are affected by, the impacts of ongoing national and local development initiatives.

Both tourists and affected national citizens need to communicate with their families, have access to information, be provided with replacement identity documentation, and be offered immediate food, drink, medical aid, and shelter. Both need to be evacuated from an affected area and then be repatriated or resettled at the earliest opportunity. As the illustration below indicates, there are numerous services and capabilities that are both shared and depended upon when responding to emergencies (see Figure 1).

While the theme *More with Less* inevitably implies achieving more with less money, it is also possible that more can be achieved with different money, less duplication, and better leadership.

The following paragraphs seek to suggest ways in which capitalizing on the needs and capabilities of travel and tourism can greatly assist national governments and international agencies in preparing for, and responding to, disasters. This chapter is by no means exhaustive and is intended to be indicative only. Furthermore, while it is recognized that terms such as "disaster," "emergency," and "crisis" are still subject to different interpretations in disaster management and travel and tourism literature, it is the purpose of this chapter to focus on the

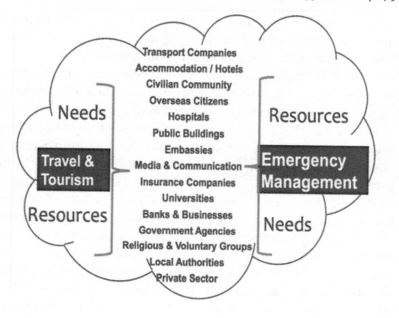

Figure 1.

unique contribution that travel and tourism can make in times of trouble.

Capitalizing on the Shared Need for National Policy

The travel and tourism industry shares with the wider international disaster management community a strong vested interest in ensuring that clear national emergency management policies exist within countries and destinations in which they operate. It is a fact that at the same time travel and tourism is experiencing significant growth, the countries that people travel to are experiencing increasing numbers of natural and man-made disasters.[12]

Many popular destinations to which tourists travel lack clear national policies for dealing with disasters. While national emergency structures and processes are continuously evolving, in many countries they remain underdeveloped and underfunded, and in some cases nonexistent. This means that the question of "Who is in charge of managing disasters?" in a given country is often not easily answered, and thus it is difficult for any key partner such as travel and tourism to integrate if clear structures do not exist or are seriously underdeveloped.

Some national governments allocate responsibility for disaster management on the basis of a recent catastrophic experience of a particular type of disaster. For example, a country that has been recently impacted by a major earthquake or flood might decide to put overall responsibility for disaster management within a Ministry of Housing (for earthquakes) or of Environment (for floods). Other governments may choose to place responsibility for managing disasters within their Ministry of Defense or within a ministry that has overall budgetary control over the emergency services, for example the Ministry of Interior, arguing that such a ministry will be better placed to deploy and resource key response assets and people in the event of all types of disaster. Still other governments have elected to create totally separate offices for disaster management, for example an "Office of the Prime Minister" or "Office of the President." They argue that a single lead ministry may lack the ability or clout to address all types of disasters whereas an office that incorporates the strengths of all ministries may be better equipped to address risk reduction, response, and recovery across all of government.

It is not the purpose of this chapter to comment on the advantages and disadvantages of the various solutions that governments have chosen to the question of who should be in charge of disaster management in any given country. Suffice it to say that "no one size fits all." What is vital, however, is that travel and tourism should participate fully in the task of advocacy for the development of such policies and plans for disasters at all levels. Dialogue with the travel and tourism industry will greatly enhance the existing work of international agencies and embassies by connecting disaster management policy directly to a country's reputation and income as a tourism destination.

Capitalizing on the Shared Need
for National Coordination

Imagine you are an ambassador living and working in a host country that is susceptible to earthquakes. Each year thousands of your own countrymen, businessmen, and tourists visit the country, spending varying lengths of time in a wide variety of locations and types of accommodation. On this day, an earthquake takes place in one of the areas of the host country in which you know that many of your national citizens routinely stay. You have no idea, of course, how many of your countrymen and women are there on this particular day. Tourists and businessmen do not routinely inform their embassies of their travel plans. You watch as the media reports rising casualty figures from scenes of devastation. What you do know is that in a very short time the Foreign Ministry back in your home country will be calling for details on how many nationals have been affected by this earthquake. Who are they? Where are they? How are they? If they are dead, have they been positively identified? If they have been evacuated to a hospital, to which hospital have they been taken? If they have been moved along with others to local or regional reception centers, to which ones have they been taken? If families have become separated in the chaos of the emergency how quickly can they be reunited? In short, "What plans are in place for locating, identifying, reuniting, and repatriating our own people?"

As ambassador you turn to your contacts in the national or local police or other emergency services to seek answers. You discover that the national and local emergency management planners have assumed that it is the task of each embassy to make contact with their own citizens for the purposes of tracking and repatriation.

However, the tasks of locating, identifying, assisting, and removing people affected by any disaster require certain core response systems that should be nationally planned for, resourced, effectively communicated, and routinely carried out, so that everyone, including embassies and the travel and tourism industry, can benefit.

Points of Liaison

First among these systems is the vital need for clear points of liaison at the national, provincial, and local levels. Clear and authoritative points of contact are required within the travel and tourism industry, with which national emergency management agencies can integrate and find a voice on behalf of the industry during emergencies. In most cases these simply do not exist. Airlines, cruise companies, hotel chains, and tour companies should create their own emergency procedures, crisis operations rooms, and methods for obtaining casualty data on their clients. However, their operations can be subsequently frustrated by decisions that are made by national, regional, and local disaster management agencies that remain unaware of the specific plans and requirements of the travel and tourism industry. As a result, for example, coaches owned and operated by a tour company, intended to take their clients from an area of danger to a place of safety, may be summarily requisitioned for government use elsewhere.

Foreign embassies and high commissions are also anxious to have clear communications and liaison with host governments to understand their emergency systems, not only to better protect their own nationals when on business trips or vacation, but also to provide effective casualty-tracking information when disasters occur.

The experience of Sri Lanka prior to, and during, the 2004 tsunami provides an excellent example of how the establishment of clear points of liaison for travel and tourism can significantly benefit disaster response.

In the years prior to the 2004 tsunami, a shared threat arising from the civil conflict in Sri Lanka had resulted in considerable collaboration between the Sri Lanka Tourism Development Authority (SLTDA) (as the lead agency for travel and tourism for the government of Sri Lanka) and the tour operators and travel companies with the common goal of operating safely in the changing security environment. An agreement was reached whereby heads of major tourist associations were required to report immediately to the SLTDA within the first hours of any crisis to report on issues affecting tourists. Three main sectors of the tourism industry were regularly represented at such meetings; these were the Tourist Hotels Association of Sri Lanka, the Travel Agents Association of Sri Lanka (for outbound tourism) and the Sri Lanka Association of Inbound Tour Operators.

On the day that the 2004 tsunami struck Sri Lanka approximately 60,000 tourists, across all nationalities, were affected. The majority of these were located within the coastal belt stretching between Matara on the south coast and Negombo on the southwest coast, north of Colombo. In accordance with previous practice, the SLTDA immediately called a crisis meeting of its members.

The Tourist Hotels Association was tasked with assessing the state of all hotels in the affected areas where most tourists were located. In particular, the requirement was to gauge the ability of hotels to continue to provide adequate food and accommodation for tourists until such time that they could be repatriated.

The Travel Agents Association of Sri Lanka was tasked with ensuring that all scheduled commercial flights to Sri Lanka should continue to arrive, but with the proviso that they be empty, thereby not adding additional tourists to the problem. It was also requested that additional empty flights be routed to Sri Lanka to assist with the repatriation task.

In addition, the SLTDA set up a command center to assist in providing additional accommodation, as well as in tracking, identifying, and evacuating all of the tourists caught up in the wake of the tsunami. A former member of the SLTDA commented after the tsunami on how important for Sri Lanka it had been that heads of tourist associations routinely gathered together in such a way immediately after a crisis: "If it had not been for our experience during the conflict we would not have got through the tsunami."[13]

A similar example of liaison for tourism during emergencies comes from Turkey. A tourism disaster platform exists which is chaired by the vice governor for tourism in Istanbul Municipality, with membership from the Ministry of Tourism, the Istanbul Hotel Association (which represents 82 percent of hotels in Istanbul which are 3-star upwards), the National Disaster Management Agency of Turkey, and representatives from the fifteen Istanbul Municipalities and the Association of Media.

Solutions for identifying national, regional, and local points of liaison for travel and tourism in a country may never be uniform. While ministries of tourism may appear an obvious first choice, their staff are mostly recruited for their skills in marketing and communication and are therefore more suited perhaps to the task of post-disaster recovery strategies to win back visitors.

An alternative approach might be for governments to draw on the experience of countries like Sri Lanka and Turkey and unite the operational and logistical skill sets of their main travel and tourism players (transportation, hotel, and tour company associations) in such a way that senior executives are brought together during emergencies to work closely alongside emergency management planners. A rotating scheme of "Duty Chief Executive" could be established so that on any given day one voice speaks for the whole travel and tourism industry at each level.

Capitalizing on the Shared Need for Effective Casualty Tracking and Information

A second core system that every nation requires is the ability to locate accurately and track disaster-affected citizens. After a disaster strikes family members are separated, work colleagues go missing, and worried relatives, at home and abroad, begin making phone calls to try and locate their loved ones. Mobile networks become overloaded as the number of calls spirals. Some people phone local hospitals but are unable to get through, as there are usually only one or two public numbers available and they will already be busy handling other callers. No one knows which hospital to call anyway, as there may be several that are handling the injured. Frustrated by the fact that they cannot get answers on the phone, worried relatives and friends may decide to travel to the affected area to continue their search in person. From an emergency-management point of view this further complicates an already difficult disaster scene, as emergency responders now have to deal with traffic congestion from people driving to the scene, thereby blocking vital routes for ambulances, fire appliances, and other emergency vehicles. Cordons will cause further frustration, as the public will not be allowed past the outer cordon and might instead start traveling to local hospitals and demanding assistance there.

Despite the fact that any national public needs to find out where and how their loved ones are after a disaster, very few countries appear to have created and resourced what might be called a "casualty tracking and information system." While numerous other emergency numbers exist, these tend to focus on calling specific emergency services to come to assist. The unique task of a casualty tracking and information system is to provide the public with a focal point to turn to in order to report their concern that a loved one is missing, and who they think may be caught up in the recent disaster. The callers are then requested to give accurate details and descriptions so that the individual can be identified. This information is then matched with information provided by the emergency services from their response to, and investigation of, the scene of the disaster. The details and descriptions of everyone who is evacuated from a disaster scene (whether injured, uninjured, or dead) or admitted to a hospital or reception center are carefully recorded and kept until a match can be made. The next of kin can be then informed that their loved one has been found and told to which reception center or hospital and ward they have been taken. In the case of a death the police will usually inform the next of kin in person.

The travel and tourism industry already recognizes the vital necessity of such a system. Operators are conscious of the impact to the reputation of their own businesses if, in the event of a disaster, they are unable to quickly and effectively answer any calls from the public regarding the location and state of health of their clients. Embassies are faced with the same urgent requirement to provide rapid information updates on who has been affected and where they are. Not to do so leads to criticism at home, ridicule in the media, and possible political damage.

Many travel and tourism companies, such as airlines, cruise companies, or tour agents, already have bespoke casualty tracking and information systems in place. They have equipped themselves to rapidly set up company call centers in the event of an emergency so that the public can have a central number to call if they are worried about a relative or friend. Other companies have contracted these services out to commercial companies who provide not only the ability to handle multiple calls from the public after a disaster, but can also handle multiple languages.

The setting up and resourcing of a national casualty tracking system need not be expensive. In countries that do have such systems police are often made responsible for providing the service. Use is made of off-duty officers or administrators to take calls from the public and to establish records of all those who have been declared as missing or likely to have been affected by the disaster. Some countries might pass this task on to other emergency services such as Civil Protection or even request assistance from their national Red Cross or Red Crescent Society.

What is vital, however, is that any and all casualty tracking and information systems should jointly establish effective liaison so as to allow accurate and timely data to be obtained and passed on to families, embassies, and other essential stakeholders. Hence, travel and tourism companies that run their own casualty tracking call centers need to find ways of sharing their data with government emergency management agencies and vice versa.

In addition to the setting up of call centers, casualty tracking also requires effective liaison between the various locations to which people are taken. In some countries, for example, hotels are connected to an online network linked to local and national police databases for the registration of guests staying in hotels. This allows emergency planners, including travel and tourism representatives, to call upon the police for details of how many tourists were staying in a given city on the day of a disaster and at which hotels.

Emergency service officers are often used to provide liaison at hospitals, reception centers, and other locations to which the injured and evacuated are taken. Their task is to help maintain accurate records of where people have been taken by being present at their admission, for example the admission of injured to a hospital, and recording those admissions in order to report back to the central casualty tracking office. Here again representatives from the travel and tourism industry could be of great assistance. Company representatives could be asked to accompany their clients to a hospital in order to track their progress and location. In addition, tourism company representatives may be among the tourists that are taken from any disaster scene to reception centers. These representatives could assist in helping to identify those people for whom they have a client responsibility and, while also passing this information on to their own organization's crisis operations room, become part of a wider network of informing embassies and national emergency responders. It is equally true, however, that tourist guides, hotel representatives, and other travel and tourism professionals may have become victims themselves.

Capitalizing on the Shared Need for Disaster Victim Identification (DVI)

Linked to casualty tracking is the task of identifying victims, including the dead. The aim of DVI is to establish the identity of every victim by comparing and matching accurate antemortem and postmortem data.

For travel and tourism, the task of DVI is essential since they have both a corporate responsibility to their clients and a business reputation to protect. Governments have a similar duty of care to their citizens and yet some continue to ignore the task of DVI, having decided that the costs of the equipment and expertise required are beyond them. DVI should be a requirement for every nation affected by disasters and is poignantly summarized by the Interpol Standing Committee on DVI as follows: "for legal, religious, cultural and other reasons, human beings have the right not to lose their identities after death."[14]

The task of gathering antemortem data can be made immeasurably easier when integrated with an effective casualty tracking system. This is because once the families and friends have reported their loved one missing and provided initial descriptions of them, they can then be contacted again to assist in the provision of antemortem data such as photographs, fingerprints, dental records, and DNA samples that can be matched with the postmortem data gathered from the scene of the disaster.

Identifying who has died is an essential part of any coroner's inquest. No death certificate can be issued to a grieving family without effective proof that the family member has actually died. Without a death certificate, life insurance policies cannot be claimed, probate cannot be applied for, and wills cannot be executed. Families are left unable to grieve properly and bring closure to their loss.

There are many challenges to DVI. Some disaster scenes can be described as "closed" in that they involve a fixed, identifiable group of people. For example, a fire in a school or office block, or a plane crash, can be described as a closed event in that, for example, the children and teachers of the school can be largely identified from prepared lists and nominal rolls. Similarly, identifying the passengers and crew killed or injured by an air crash can be assisted by an aircraft manifest. An "open" event, on the other hand, involves a disaster scene where there is no simple way of limiting who may have been affected. Train or bus accidents, terrorist attacks on restaurants or nightclubs, earthquakes or storm surges on densely populated areas, and even panic stampedes at religious or pop festivals are all notoriously difficult open events. Affected people could include local inhabitants, visiting friends and relatives, external contractors or businessmen and, of course, national and international tourists.

To overcome the cost of developing an in-house capability for DVI, travel companies, particularly airlines, employ the services of professional DVI organizations and pay a retainer so that they can call on their services in time of need. These services, when called upon, are often paid for through insurance taken out for such eventualities. Governments often adopt a similar strategy by retaining a professional DVI company in order to create an immediate national DVI capability. In due course they may choose to develop the skills required to manage and maintain their own national DVI teams. Some countries are looking to require commercial industries, for example mineral, chemical, oil, building, and transportation companies including rail, road, tunnel, air, and sea, to contribute to a national insurance premium to help cover the task of DVI activities in the event of major incidents causing loss of life.

Capitalizing on Travel and Tourism's Transportation, Food, and Shelter Assets

Travel and tourism incorporates services and industries that provide transportation, accommodation, and eating and drinking. While all of these services are vital components of any disaster relief effort, the fact that they usually sit within the private sector means that they are not directly under the control of the government and its emergency services. This means that their involvement in any response has to be pre-planned and agreed upon in order for it to be effective.

For example, almost every disaster response requires transportation to assist in evacuation, relief supplies, and logistical support. National emergency management agencies are not intended to be transportation companies with their own fleets of coaches, trucks, and drivers. Instead, most sign memoranda of understanding with commercial bus or lorry companies for their fleets to be called upon during times of emergency. The principle behind this approach is important to achieving more with less.

Disaster management should not be about creating huge and expensive organizations requiring unsustainable funding in order to have "under command" all of the assets that they may require during an emergency. Instead, the skill of effective disaster management is to first identify every possible existing response capacity. Then it becomes necessary, through effective communication and leadership, to secure the support and participation of the owners of those assets to assist in an integrated response when called upon.

Some countries employ legislation to enforce their requirement for certain assets when they are required. While commandeering may be effective, the old English adage "a volunteer is worth twenty pressed men" is still true. Voluntary organizations such as the British Virgin Islands Search and Rescue organization (VISAR) continue to demonstrate the potential of winning hearts and minds to assist in times of emergency as opposed to merely seeking to enforce their cooperation. Whether volunteered or commandeered, transportation still requires effective coordination.

The travel and tourism sector can also assist by providing food and shelter to affected people. During the response to the tsunami in 2004 the Sri Lanka Tourist Board negotiated an agreement with the Bandaranaike Memorial International Conference Hall (BMICH) to use its meeting rooms to provide shelter for people displaced by the disaster. Food and drink were provided by the catering franchise from the Mount Lavinia Hotel. The Sri Lanka Tourist Board accepted financial responsibility for compensating both BMICH and the Mount Lavinia Hotel catering company.

A second example of the wider provision of food and accommodation, from the 2011 earthquake and tsunami in eastern Japan, demonstrates that early warning systems and procedures adopted by emergency planners can also have knock-on effects for affected citizens; nevertheless these knock-on effects can be ameliorated by an engagement with the wider travel and tourism industry.

When the first seismic waves of the 2011 earthquake were detected in Japan, an early warning system automatically activated emergency brakes stopping a total of twenty-seven high-speed trains (Shinkansen) who were at that time traveling at maximum speeds of 330 kilometers per hour. While the automatic train control system undoubtedly saved lives, the suspension of rail operations presented another problem for emergency responders. Hundreds of thousands of commuters were now faced with no way of returning to their homes and were in need of shelter and food. Many hotels now opened their doors to invite evacuees to stay inside. The Metropolitan Hotel, for example, invited the public into the hotel lobby, banquet rooms, restaurants, hallway, and stairs for an overnight stay. They provided commuters with blankets and sheets, hot tea, power chargers for their mobile phones, and provided them with updated information on the recommencement of public transport services. The hotel also sent a voluntary team of restaurant staff to Tohoku to prepare and serve meals to evacuees staying in shelters.[15] All of this activity was done on a voluntary basis, without any mention of such provision being mentioned in their corporate emergency management manuals. The principle is striking.

Capitalizing on the Shared Need for Risk Reduction

Travel and tourism, like any industry wishing to invest capital and resources in a country, demands confidence from the point of view of
its shareholders and clients. The industry is thus a key stakeholder in
ensuring that a government takes seriously the task of risk reduction
across all of its hazards, natural and man-made. Vulnerability to risk is
often more about the decisions made by government regarding its citizens than the physical hazards it faces.

Like all industries, travel and tourism can have both a positive and
negative impact on a country. Tourism can, for example, uniquely enhance the physical and cultural qualities of a community while also
using them for profit. It can also, however, cause damage to local ecosystems and the community culture, and contribute to pollution and
global warming. Furthermore, it can be a competitor for scarce resources and aggravate a destination's vulnerability to hazards by
creating an unsuitable physical infrastructure and encouraging an
unsustainable influx of workers. It is therefore vital that the travel and
tourism industry be fully integrated into any risk reduction strategy at
all levels.

At the UN conference on environment and development held in Rio
de Janeiro in June 1992 (the Rio Earth Summit), 180 countries adopted
"Agenda 21" which sought to establish sustainable international development practices while maintaining the integrity of the global environment.[16] In 1995 UNWTO, in collaboration with the World Travel
and Tourism Council, produced their own revised version of Agenda 21
in order to encourage sustainable tourism.[17] They defined sustainable
tourism as: "Tourism that takes full account of its current and future
economic, social and environmental impacts, addressing the needs of
the visitors, the industry, the environment and host communities," and
argued that sustainable tourism:

• should not adversely affect the environment;

• should be acceptable to the community;

- should be profitable for businesses;

- should satisfy the visitor.

While these aims have been adopted by some travel and tourism organizations, there is some cynicism from governments, tourism professionals, and consumers as to the practicality of implementing them from a financial viewpoint. The need to generate employment and income from the travel and tourism of 980 million visitors will inevitably have impacts globally.

There is now a new urgency for sustainable tourism development driven in part by climate change, the expected growth in travel and tourism by 2025, and the number of disasters around the world that are closely linked to tourism and its development.

While national legislatures make regulations on land use and governments offer economic incentives such as tax exemption for projects that encourage positive, safe, and sustainable tourism development, pressures continue to emerge from the travel and tourist industry to allow developments which sow the seeds of future risk. The development of holiday destinations in coastal resorts at risk of tsunamis, hotel complexes in seismically active areas, or demands for the removal of natural barriers to sea surges and hurricanes in order to reclaim land for tourism conflict with the objectives of sustainable development. In this respect the travel and tourism development agenda can be part of the problem of risk in a country, and it is vital that their agenda be incorporated within a wider risk reduction strategy.

Efficient and effective disaster reduction, and adaptation to climate change, requires the involvement of all stakeholders in sharing interests and knowledge and cooperating closely in developing common standards and investing in common solutions. The travel and tourism industry often presents a fragmented front and requires central coordination and integration at both community and national levels in order to play an effective role in sustainable development.

There are obvious questions to which travel and tourism, along with other agencies, can contribute answers in order to have up-to-date information and analysis on international, national, and local hazards affecting the areas in which they operate.

Such questions include:

- What are the likely hazards that affect these areas?

- Are the hazards seasonal or difficult/impossible to predict?

- In what ways are the affected population (and therefore tourists) vulnerable to these hazards?

- Have these hazards been mapped (either with a geographic information system [GIS] or on more traditional hazard maps) and by whom?

- Are these maps available to the travel and tourism industry or have they been unnecessarily over classified as "confidential" or "secret"?

- Are the national and local emergency services fully aware of the potential impact of these hazards on tourist populations vacationing in the areas at risk?

- Are the national and local government agencies fully aware of the risks to the livelihoods of local communities, for whom tourism is the main economic activity, if hazards are insufficiently managed?

Ministries of tourism can also assist in the analysis of trends in tourism development in areas of risk. They could, for example, help avoid dangerous developments by requiring destination developers and builders to maintain strict building codes and land-use management. In addition, they could help assess the capacity of operators such as cruise companies with ships operating in regions where an evacuation from a ship onto a nearby island could overwhelm the facilities available. Other areas where travel and tourism could contribute in risk reduction include the development of effective early warning systems, shared hazard mapping projects, and shared simulations and exercises.

Capitalizing on the Shared Need for Recovery

The theme of this chapter has been restricted to preparing for, and responding to, disasters. Nevertheless, a brief mention must be made too of the economic, social, and environmental contribution that the industry can make to the speed and depth of recovery after a disaster.

It seems to be widely understood that travel and tourism can bring much-needed income after disaster strikes. Ministries of tourism create campaigns to encourage tourists to return to the region. For example, after Hurricane Katrina devastated New Orleans the New Orleans Convention and Visitors Bureau created a visitor campaign called "Forever New Orleans." As a result the Mardi Gras of 2007 saw visitor numbers rise to 800,000, which gave the city a welcome $20 million in tax revenues to help in the recovery of the economy, and in 2009 these numbers successfully reverted back to the pre-Katrina figure of 1 million visitors.

What appears less well appreciated is the fact that tourism can also help to rebuild national life at the community level. In 2005, for example, tourists voluntarily traveled to Sri Lanka to offer their services in rebuilding local communities and infrastructure. Such "voluntourism" attracts those who are already interested in the people, arts, culture, geography, heritage sites, and natural environment of a country to volunteer their skills, as their holiday, and to serve and enhance the destination. Similarly, in 2005, after Hurricane Katrina had devastated New Orleans, many traveled to the city to see the devastation for themselves and stayed to assist the local community. To encourage this activity, tour operators and a major hotel chain in New Orleans offered a package called "Spirit to Serve New Orleans" which included the opportunity to work on a voluntary basis with the New Orleans Area Habitat for Humanity or the Second Harvest Food Bank of New Orleans.

The fact that skilled people wish to make themselves available, and at no cost, is a powerful argument for ensuring that this unique form of tourism is both encouraged and coordinated. As with all external assistance, however, the arrival of individuals or teams of volunteer helpers requires careful integration and coordination to ensure that the end results meet desired objectives.

Capitalizing on Travel and Tourism: Conclusions

In this chapter I have sought to highlight some of the many ways in which travel and tourism can assist in preparing for and responding to disasters. Sadly, in many countries, the industry continues to be side-lined or ignored. This chapter concludes with some general observations as to the likely barriers to capitalizing on the industry in preparing for and responding to disasters.

Mutual understanding. There is still a widespread lack of dialogue between national emergency planning agencies and the travel and tourism industry. Appropriate structures and points of liaison are needed if the industry is to effectively integrate its contribution to reducing risk and responding to disasters. Each national government should ensure that there is a clear and authoritative lead for travel and tourism so that the industry is properly represented within the emergency management structures at each level of national coordination. Emergency management agencies need to develop an understanding of travel and tourism as a victim, and also as part of their solutions. At the same time, travel and tourism needs to understand the systems and objectives of disaster management within the countries in which they operate. They will then be able to better ensure that their needs can be met and their contribution properly integrated.

Smaller is acceptable. There is a tendency in lesser-developed countries for the international community to encourage the creation of expensive and manpower-intensive structures for national disaster management. While such solutions provide much-needed employment, they also create considerable funding dependencies. Some national disaster management budget requirements appear larger than those required by their government colleagues for routine governance. To achieve more with less requires a greater awareness of what others can provide and a more open and facilitative attitude toward integration.

Ownership versus leadership. Effective disaster management should be more about leadership than ownership. National disaster management ministries and agencies tend to prefer organigrams that show all assets, capabilities, and stakeholders linked with an unbroken line of command and control. Disaster management directors need to provide leadership and communication skills to win the hearts and minds of organizations, both public and private, who can contribute but are not mandated to do so.

Duplication versus collaboration. There is a need to avoid duplication. In recent years there has been an explosion in the growth of crisis operations rooms and information systems across ministries, agencies, and private sector companies. Ways must now be found to share information between private and public sector agencies during a crisis. Issues of confidentiality and security must be addressed while also ensuring that information centers do not become "sinks" of data but rather active shared hubs. Decision-makers need to be able to observe and orientate to facts on the ground in order to conduct effective situational analysis and make decisions for action. Senior executives can be lured into believing that costly networks of CCTV cameras with uplinks to crisis operations rooms, manned twenty-four hours a day, provide all the necessary situational awareness required to respond effectively in times of crisis. Images on CCTV screens may be meaningless, however, if not accompanied by local comment from relevant observers on the ground, which provides the context. Similarly, since many public and private organizations have developed GIS mapping databases of their activities it makes sense for emergency planners to negotiate access to specific data owned by such organizations rather than create duplicate (or conflicting) versions of the same data on their separate databases.

Lessons identified versus lessons learned. Finally, there is a continuing need to learn from the lessons identified from previous crises. Reports written after disaster events highlight what happened and what went wrong. However, lessons that are identified need then to be translated into lessons learned, and it is here that progress must be made to avoid costly repeats of the same mistakes. Changes in senior personnel often mean that lessons are forgotten as a result of a lack of sufficient handover training to successor appointments. Joint exercises to test integrated plans are regarded with suspicion and fear by senior executives within public and private agencies who worry that the exercise may reveal any lack of ability in themselves or their organization. In order to overcome this fear integrated exercises of crisis plans are often reduced to mere organization drills of previously identified actions at a specifically agreed date and time.

Business in an Age of Emergency

RICHARD BRANSON

Businesses have always had a role in helping communities during tough times and especially in response to disasters. After all, business would not exist without its communities. So when tornados, earthquakes, hurricanes, fires, or tsunamis strike, businesses must do their part.

Companies small and large can and often do step into the breach to do whatever they can in the wake of disaster. Many businesses have services and products that can help with relief efforts, and all have communities and networks they can work with to raise awareness and much needed funds during an emergency. During any disaster response, pharmaceutical companies provide antibiotics, vitamins, medicine, and water purification tablets; telecoms offer text-to-donate capabilities and emergency communication support; distributors and transporters get food, medicine, and shelter to the affected people; banks offer matching grants and cash-for-work voucher assistance; construction companies provide labor, materials, and equipment; health-care providers sponsor emergency physicians and medical assistance. The list of private sector contributions goes on and on.

Obviously this is good. Governments, nongovernmental organizations (NGOs), and local communities need help when disaster strikes. We're fortunate across the Virgin Group that we've got businesses in over fifteen different industries we can rally for support. Virgin responds to many disasters with as much support as possible, but we all must do more. In the last ten years, I have watched more disasters strike with a devastating human toll than in the previous thirty combined. I have come to believe that this is not an anomaly, but a new normal. We've entered an "Age of Emergency," and it is related to many big trends: rapid urbanization and population growth have put billions more in harm's way; climate change is leading to more uncertain and violent weather; and resource scarcity could lead us into a new era of tension and man-made crisis.

Fortunately, for the first time in history, our newly connected world is better equipped to respond to disasters and mobilize global support. Now all we need to do is ensure we effectively coordinate and collaborate, bringing together the best of the business, social, and governmental sectors. Business also has a significant responsibility to help stop some of the emergencies from happening in the first place, for example by reversing trends like climate change and the degradation of our natural resources. The private sector should get serious about understanding the causes and consequences of disasters and playing a role in all phases of a crisis.

The Age of Emergency Is upon Us

The increasing destruction caused by natural disasters is mind-blowing. In the past decade, 3,800 disasters occurred and killed more than 780,000 people around the world. Over 2 billion people were affected—this averages to more than 250 million people a year. These extreme events have touched every corner of the globe and have cost the international community close to $960 billion.[1]

Earthquakes are now killing more people than ever in urban areas where buildings are not properly designed. More people live on coasts, and as climate change raises sea levels and increases the ferocity of storms, they will be on the edge of disaster. Many countries are increasing their reliance on nuclear power, with the risk of Fukushima-type disasters with long-term consequences.

On top of these natural disasters, our global village continues to suffer from violent conflicts that become even greater emergencies when coupled with natural disasters such as drought. In Somalia, recent droughts caused tens of thousands of deaths and created millions of refugees. The United Nations High Commissioner for Refugees (UNHCR) reported that Dadaab, the world's largest refugee camp in neighboring Kenya, swelled to over 460,000 people as a result.[2] The vicious cycle of conflict and emergency can be unstoppable. Security threats from refugee flows, for example, lead regional security forces to enter into battle with rebel forces, driving even more displacement, causing more suffering, and disrupting relief efforts. Much of this could have been avoided if the world acted more effectively to stave off conflict and respond rapidly to new emergencies. Businesses, governments, and the social sector must start to coordinate—not only to respond to emergencies, but also to proactively forecast emergencies and try to stop them.

In short, we have entered the Age of Emergency, and for businesses everywhere, recognizing this change and responding to it will be one of the imperatives for success in the coming years.

The resources to help populations hit by disaster come through a chaotic and complicated web of actors. First, and with primary responsibility, are the governments of the countries hit by disaster and the major international relief agencies in the United Nations (UN) like the World Food Programme, the United Nations Children's Fund, UNHCR, and the Food and Agricultural Organization (FAO), along with the International Committee of Red Cross and Red Crescent, which have humanitarian responsibilities under international law. Then there are countless national aid agencies like Department for International Development (DFID) in the UK and the United States Agency for International Development (USAID). Local and international NGOs like Oxfam, CARE, and Save the Children, religious relief organizations like Catholic Relief Services and World Vision, and thousands of private foundations are the next major players, often doing what governments and aid agencies cannot or will not do. And finally, the private sector—businesses themselves, not just their foundations or philanthropic arms—play a vital role, mainly as donors of supplies, expertise, and resources. The UN Office for the Coordination of Humanitarian Affairs (OCHA) is supposed to coordinate and integrate among all of these actors, and is helped by coordinating bodies like Interaction and AmeriCares in the United States.

The private sector is vital to helping innocent people get through extraordinarily difficult circumstances during a crisis and pressing governments to be proactive. The victims of disasters need the world with them, and every government hit with a tragedy needs help. In 2009, the foreign minister of Pakistan visited me during the UN General Assembly in New York. He described the flooding in Pakistan in the most clear and compelling terms. Close to 20 million people were affected. Hundreds of miles of roads and bridges were wiped out. Farms were flooded. Children were stranded. Local governments were underwater and unable to help their people. Because the media wasn't able to get out to the remote areas, it took a while for people to realize how significant this catastrophe was. One-fifth of Pakistan was under water. Tents, food, clean water, and medicine were needed.

The business community reached out. My foundation, Virgin Unite, hosted a fundraiser. Cash contributions, matching donations, warehousing support, medical supplies, and food came into the country from companies like Abbott, Bank of America, BP, Cargill, Cisco, GE, Google, Kraft Foods, Microsoft, Pfizer, Procter and Gamble, UPS, and Western Union.

But governments do not always reach out like this or respond well, and politics can cost lives. During the devastating cyclone in Myanmar most international relief organizations faced restricted access because the military leaders feared international scrutiny. Visas were denied. While the international community waited for permits and landing permissions, aid trickled in slowly, harming tens of thousands of homeless and injured victims.

In a humanitarian crisis there is no room for politics. That includes the private sector. Everything is interrelated. Business needs government and the social sector. Government and the social sector need business. And communities need us to work together.

Governments need to include the private sector in disaster response programming and the private sector needs to step up to the plate and take responsibility for our global village. Everyone is scrambling to find their place in the immediate aftermath of a crisis. Everyone is aiming to be first with the most. But there are problems inherent with lots of actors. Lots of money leads to lots of corruption and lots of waste. Too much is spent on immediate emergency response, too little on longer-term recovery, and scandalously little on preparation and prevention that could save countless lives before disaster strikes.

Having helped out in dozens of crises, both man-made and natural, I have come to believe that the magnitude of destruction we now see requires *greater involvement from the private sector in every phase of a disaster*. To think about this whole ecosystem of disaster relief and how business fits into it, it helps to consider our role as it is now in each phase of a disaster and how we might change to be more effective. We need to consider our role and what we could do better in *emergency response and relief*; *recovery and reconstruction*; and *preparation and risk mitigation*. Finally, in the larger context of a world with ever more disasters striking ever more people, businesses need to think about the *bigger picture* and *the systemic challenges* that have brought us to the Age of Emergency.

Emergency Response and Relief

We wake up to the images of devastation. Whole villages and towns washed away by the Indian Ocean tsunami, the capital of Haiti flattened, New Orleans under water, fires or mudslides carrying people to their graves, a nuclear reactor melting down in Japan. At these moments, common humanity trumps everything and we all respond. From school kids to Fortune 500 corporations, we're at our best in the immediate aftermath of tragedy. Like many private companies, the Virgin Group looks to its core competencies, its presence and relationships in the affected area, and its network to see what we can do to help. The Virgin Emergency Response team draws on a network of contacts across the Virgin Group and relevant outside partners that can move quickly to support global emergencies. Over the years, we've learned a whole lot about what has worked, and what hasn't.

One of the assets we can mobilize quickly in times of disaster is our planes. All of our airlines, from Virgin Atlantic to Virgin Australia, have been incredibly generous at times of great disaster. In 1998, Virgin Atlantic operated a relief flight into the Caribbean, carrying 27 tons of supplies to help islanders affected by Hurricane Georges. In 2005, when Pakistan suffered a devastating earthquake, Virgin Atlantic dispatched an aid flight with 55 tons of aid including tents, tarpaulin, plastic sheeting, children's clothing, and Shelterboxes. In 2004, when hundreds of thousands of people had been washed away and millions more were in danger after the Indian Ocean tsunami, we coordinated with other industry leaders to fill two Virgin Atlantic planes with lifesaving supplies within a day of the crisis. We also raised money for the Disasters Emergency Committee through our Change for Children onboard collection drive and launched a campaign across all Virgin businesses globally to raise funds and awareness.

We've also worked with our airlines to help countries facing war and conflict. In 1990, Virgin flew into Iraq to operate aid flights and operated the only hostage-release flight from Baghdad. After the 2003 U.S.-led invasion of Iraq, we had a lot of Iraqi citizens contacting us to see if we could get urgent medical supplies to Basra and the British military looking for humanitarian assistance and help with the airport. My team mobilized close to 60 tons of medical supplies worth more than £2 million/$3 million from dozens of pharmaceutical companies and partners. We filled our plane. And along with some Iraqi doctors, we flew Virgin Atlantic to Basra. We were the first relief flight into Iraq, and we found a dire situation.

I'll never forget the devastating feeling of walking into a hospital in Basra where children torn apart by the bombs and bullets did not even have access to painkillers. I was relieved that our shipment would provide some temporary relief, but daunted by the sheer scale of the need. It was a turning point for me, and when I got back to London I made sure that the Virgin Group organized across our 300 businesses to collaborate in times of disaster. We started then to work more closely with governments and the social sector to respond more effectively as a global village. We continue to work daily to help governments and aid agencies be prepared.

We are also learning from the great work that other businesses are doing. For example, companies like Coca-Cola leverage their massive distribution networks—which reach literally into almost every community on earth—to deliver aid from hubs like airports rapidly to affected areas. Large retailers like Target partner with official emergency management agencies to ensure they have support and supplies to respond quickly in the event of a disaster and help raise public awareness about disaster preparedness. And of course, businesses can mobilize cash, probably the most important contribution during a disaster. When historic floods hit Queensland, Australia, all five major Virgin companies there, as well as Virgin Unite, stepped up to raise money and awareness.

There are problems with everyone doing much at the same time in the early days after a disaster. More aid often arrives than can be effectively managed and distributed. Corruption and scams divert resources intended for victims. And often, the aid received is not what is most needed. Transparency International and other organizations have done some good work on analyzing and understanding corruption in disaster response. We need to strike a balance—too great a focus on corruption could lead to paralysis and itself delay vital assistance. So a risk management framework should be adopted and we in the private sector can hopefully help develop that framework. We always look at and manage risks to our businesses, be it from waste, theft, and fraud or from competition. Business practices could help aid coordinating organizations like OCHA and Interaction better manage risk and help the right assistance reach the right people.

The earthquake that struck Haiti in 2010 was the worst in two centuries, and it hit people living and working in buildings that had no proper design for earthquake safety. Three hundred thousand died and 1.5 million were left homeless. I was in my home on Necker Island at the time. I remember getting a call from Jean Oelwang, the CEO of Virgin Unite. The devastation on the television was heartbreaking and I was proud to see that Virgin Unite and companies throughout the Virgin Group were moving into emergency response before I made my first call.

As always, the first seventy-two hours were all about saving lives. Money poured in. Aid agencies and governments from around the world sent helicopters and lifesaving support. Virgin Unite kicked off a major campaign across the Virgin businesses. Virgin Atlantic and Virgin America planes flew tents, blankets, cookware, toiletries, and water filtration equipment to Miami for distribution. We also offered cargo and passenger space to injured Haitians and to international relief staff based in London, Miami, Orlando, and Jamaica. Again, our onboard passenger appeal kicked into action raising funds right away for Change for Children and many of our other businesses launched campaigns to raise awareness and funds. After our first phase, Virgin Unite joined with the Reuben Foundation to hold major fundraisers in London to support Free the Children and we were able to assist efforts like the SOS Children's Villages that acted as a base camp for emergency relief and a refuge for orphaned and homeless children. These funds also supported the many schools, clinics and sanitation facilities established by Free the Children.

But six months after the Haiti earthquake, the television cameras were mostly gone and the surge was subsiding. The international community took stock: 10 million cubic feet of rubble, a slow and stubborn cholera epidemic. An astonishing 5,000 NGOs had sprung up and political infighting and corruption were slowing the move toward recovery. Two years after the earthquake, only about half the rubble is gone and just over half the $4.5 billion pledged by the world for recovery has been disbursed.[3] A half million Haitians remain homeless.[4]

Many observers have noted that the vast majority of aid comes in the first two months after a disaster; one-third in the first few weeks alone. Fewer realize how dramatically the assistance drops off and that "giving stops almost completely after five or six months."[5]

If enough funds are available, slowing and drawing out spending can be a good thing, ensuring that there are funds to support lifting the country out of disaster. We need to get to a point where post-disaster relief sparks reconstruction and leads to hope and economic gain for the local populace. This should be based on empowerment of the local population and local institutions, but according to a recent report, only 6 percent of foreign aid to Haiti goes through local institutions.[6] People sometimes call Haiti the "Republic of NGOs," which is both good—there is some absolutely heroic and effective work being done through local and international collaboration—and worrying because people need to transition to something more sustainable than international aid.

The best examples build in the transition from response to recovery. Paul Farmer and Partners In Health (PIH) have made a huge difference to lives in Haiti, reaching tens of thousands with quality, timely medical care. By creating a national teaching hospital and focusing on building survivors' skills through the Stand with Haiti fund, PIH was able to scale up partnerships with local communities who will then have the capabilities to continue to provide care long after the international community has flown out.

But when I look at Haiti today, I think that we in the international private sector have missed an opportunity to move from emergency response to recovery. Ironically, this is where doing good and doing well can best come together. As societies get past the relief stage, business opportunities should become the first priority, and international partnerships and investment are possible catalysts for more sustainable recovery than ongoing aid and NGO efforts.

Preparation and Risk Mitigation

Despite the staggering death tolls, the grimmest natural disaster statistic is this: around 85 percent of those exposed to risks from earthquakes, cyclones, floods, and droughts live in developing countries.[7] Already fragile, these populations face greater risk than their more well-off neighbors. Disasters can literally wipe out low-income societies merely because they are unprepared. According to the UN, "if a cyclone of the same magnitude were to strike both Japan and the Philippines, mortality in the Philippines would be 17 times higher. Yet Japan has 1.4 times more people exposed to tropical cyclones than the Philippines. The mortality risk for equal numbers of people exposed in low income countries is nearly 200 times higher than in OECD countries."[8]

An ounce of basic risk reduction will be worth a pound of emergency response and relief in developing countries. We all know that the Haiti earthquake did not need to kill so many people. Yet organizations across all sectors are less likely to focus on prevention than on disaster relief. Tragically, the private sector tends to do business as usual, sticking only to minimum standards to maximize profits. Of course governments are responsible for the regulations and enforcement of standards like building codes to ensure more people live through a natural calamity. But many governments that are struggling with dire poverty and conflict are unable to take on this role. The private sector can do more. Just waiting for governments to get their act together is a cop-out and not very smart from a business perspective. I believe that companies that guarantee higher standards and challenge governments to regulate well rather than exploit loopholes will do better over time.

Whether in China where scandalously poor school construction cost the lives of thousands of children in the Chengdu earthquake in 2008 or in the Philippines where towns continue to expand into areas with endemic mudslides, the private sector can be a part of driving better standards. This can be done very publicly. Highlighting for customers—from individual homeowners to corporations to governments—how other companies fail to do things right and how committing to higher standards will generate new business and brand loyalty and can give forward-thinking companies a competitive edge. Many states reeling from the costs of a disaster will look to rebuild better, and companies with a track record of high standards will be positioned to gain these contracts. The markets will side with businesses that do good in addition to doing well when it comes to things like safer construction.

The best response to any disaster is being prepared. We should refuse to accept the unacceptable fact that billions live at unnecessary risk. With governments failing to step up, the private sector should collaborate with disaster response and prevention experts to identify best practices and standards for everything from construction to advance planning and pre-positioning of critical supplies like medicine and clean water to consequence management for dangerous materials released in an earthquake, flood, or tsunami.

We also need to work together to predict emergencies and take action before they even get started. Droughts and food emergencies are often "slow-moving" and have predictable consequences. In Somalia, for example, it was very clear that drought would push the already dire situation over the edge and leave thousands of people starving, which is exactly what happened in 2010. All of us could have worked together to help ensure that steps were taken to prevent and respond to the crisis in advance. Clarity about impending human crises could have sparked new initiatives to rally support to the beleaguered transitional government in place in Somalia. But as former FAO head Jose Graziano da Silva recently wrote, "the Horn of Africa has suffered three droughts, followed by severe crises. Each time, the international community agreed that long-term measures were needed to prevent another tragedy. But each time, when the rains finally came, the world's good intentions melted away." Forward-thinking businesses can help us break this unfortunate cycle and start getting ahead of emergencies.

The Bigger Picture

We have not come into an Age of Emergency by chance. According to the Global Humanitarian Forum, a reasonable estimate is to attribute 40 percent of the increase in natural disasters since 1980 to climate change.[9] My work with Virgin Unite in creating the Carbon War Room has only reinforced my belief that unless we focus on systemic problems, we will only continue to face disaster and response, a vicious cycle that will leave us little time for developing the world we all want to leave to our children. Businesses have played a large role in the degradation of natural resources that have led to climate change, and must play a role in getting us back on course. My work with the Elders, an initiative incubated by Virgin Unite, has also shown me the significant role that conflict has in catalyzing and continuing emergencies.

The world is becoming one in which the business community has to work closely with governments in helping them get a lot of problems resolved. It's up to business to innovate, to come up with fuels that can power our planes that emit lower levels of carbon, with ways of utilizing the sun and the wind at a fraction of what it currently costs. I'm a strong believer that business should be a force for good, not just a moneymaking machine for its shareholders. Governments and businesses have the opportunity to work together to build the right market conditions that will stimulate the use of renewable fuels and help stop the destruction of our natural assets. Jochen Zeitz from PUMA, just launched an initiative that fully values the use of natural assets on their balance sheet. Can you imagine what a different world we would live in if every business were to do this kind of environmental profit and loss?

With the Carbon War Room, we bring together entrepreneurs and harness their energy and resources to bring to scale market-based approaches to carbon reduction. The idea is to use the carrot much more than the stick to work with industries into trying to get gigatons (billions of tons) of carbon out of industries. It's hopefully going to make your industry more profitable and help avert disasters ahead from the lack of natural resources and increasing global warming. More independent coordinating bodies like the Carbon War Room and the Elders need to help tackle some of the tougher global issues we are facing.

Where We Go Now

We at Virgin are advocates of the idea that business can and must make a difference. When a disaster strikes, we recognize that governments and NGOs cannot do it alone. Simply getting food, water, medicine, and tents to needed populations is a challenge. Significant relief efforts require the support of businesses. We need improvements in at least three areas: bridging the public–private divide in all phases of disaster response and disaster risk management; focusing private capabilities on prevention; and shifting to sustainable, economic models for both recovery and prevention that are anchored in business and private enterprise. For each of these, the private sector can take action.

Public–Private Coordination

OCHA coordinates and tracks humanitarian assistance through its Consolidated Appeals Process (CAP). Building on OCHA and its rather strong financial tracking system to include and incorporate business would be a good start. UN, government, and NGO agencies are all more involved with this coordination than the private sector, and although OCHA is stepping up its outreach to businesses, much more could be done.

Many in the private sector do not know who to coordinate with or how. But in a situation where there is a natural disaster, we need close collaboration more than ever. We've worked with the Disaster Emergency Committee, an alliance of thirteen UK charities associated with disaster-related issues such as providing clean water, humanitarian aid, and medical care. In the aftermath of the 2004 Indian Ocean tsunami, the DEC provided 3,000 telephone lines for people to give donations and ran television campaigns in order to obtain donations. It was instrumental in coordinating the efforts of the member charities so that all the areas affected received aid and that there was no overlap in the services provided in any one area.

Think about how this kind of coordination is not connected to the coordination of governments and international organizations. When we don't collaborate or be responsible, business and governments can do harm by doing good.

Wouldn't it be much more efficient if we had preventive disaster mechanisms in place? From a business perspective, it raises many questions. When a natural disaster occurs, is there a rapid reaction from the business community that rallies around government and the NGOs and mobilizes resources? Is there a constant commitment by the business community to bear witness to all the tragedies in the world and do good? As every disaster needs action, so do the rolling crises that receive little attention. It is tragic that aid per tsunami victim was over $3,000 but victims of floods in Mozambique saw only $120 per victim.[10]

Virgin will continue to urge our private sector counterparts to band together and form a coalition to work with the UN, governments, and NGOs. Together we may be able to start a coordinated private sector counterpart to the OCHA structures like the Inter-Agency Standing Committee that coordinates public assistance and gives the international community a single point of entry for large businesses and industry in disaster relief and recovery.

Prevention

We need to change the way we approach a crisis. It's not that businesses can do it better; it's that we should tackle the crisis as a holistic community, working with NGOs and government in one collective voice. In addition to institutionalizing private sector participation and creating clear channels for collaboration, the business community needs to make risk reduction a key element of doing business. We need to help stop future natural disasters from causing the kind of apocalyptic tragedy that we have seen in recent years.

I think the business community can band together to make sustainable long-term commitments to better standards and investments in risk reduction to make the world much safer. We need to make the corporate community more robust and efficient to meet the challenges. I started my foundation Virgin Unite to help tackle some of the world's toughest problems—to see how we could use our skills across Virgin Group to help create lasting, entrepreneurial approaches to some of these devastating issues. I run Virgin Unite just as I would any other business, making sure that our investments have the best possible social and environmental return. Money is often the least important bit—what matters is that people are figuring out ways to use the assets of their businesses to drive not only profits, but progress toward a better world.

As I described in my book, *Screw Business as Usual*, I think we can make the world better just by doing things differently—and this is a key means by which we can change the way we do business to make a difference. For example, most of us have continuity of operations planning for our businesses to help us weather disasters. We should start to incorporate disaster response and risk mitigation planning for the community and victims of disasters into these efforts.

Anchoring Recovery

When we start a new venture at Virgin, we base it on hard research and analysis. Typically, we review the industry and put ourselves in the customer's shoes to see what could make it better. We ask fundamental questions: Is this an opportunity for restructuring a market and creating competitive advantage? What are the competitors doing? Is the customer confused or badly served? Is this an opportunity for building the Virgin brand? Can we add value? Will it interact with our other businesses? Is there an appropriate tradeoff between risk and reward?

One of the great failures in international aid programs is that they do not start with the same kind of questions. They are dependent on an infusion of international money, partners, and incentives, and they rarely put themselves in the shoes of their "customers," the victims of disasters receiving assistance. Of course this is not surprising because, unlike customers, aid recipients are not the source of resources for aid agencies. But asking the kinds of questions businesses ask can help relief empower people to go from being victims back to citizens and, yes, customers. I think this is the main reason international aid generally fails to transition into local and economically self-sustaining activities. Businesses can play an anchoring role by partnering their assets with communities, finding opportunities, and growing local industry and employment.

Crisis to Action

This is the decade in which we together will decide how to face an Age of Emergency. More disasters will come, millions more will be affected, and it seems like many—in governments, NGOs, international organizations, and the private sector—recognize that we need a new framework to act in concert to avoid calamity.

The challenges come at many levels—from coordinating assistance in the tortured days right after a disaster to getting serious about recovery and investing in preventive measures that can help break the cycle of crisis and suffering. While looking at all of this, we must not forget to act to reverse and mitigate the impact of the destruction of our natural assets and resulting climate change, as it conspires with population growth and overcrowding to make each disaster worse for more innocent people.

Innovations today give us great cause for hope. With text messaging and technologies like Global Positioning System (GPS) and Google maps being woven together, and with online information-clearing houses like ReliefWeb and CAP, everyone responding to a crisis has better real-time information. The OpenStreetMap process in post-earthquake Haiti allowed existing public maps, declassified government satellite imagery, private sector imagery, and information gathered by everyone from the World Bank to small local NGOs to build a living picture of the post-quake environment. These new technologies are making previously unimagined collaborations possible from relief through recovery.

The private sector needs to step up and revamp its approach to play a part in driving innovation in this Age of Emergency. This includes the Virgin Group. We need to pay more attention to recovery and prevention. Governments and NGOs need to embrace us and help us learn how to understand and positively impact every phase of every disaster. As we absorb the lessons from the last decade and come together around the technology and innovations that are helping us respond, I am sure we will all come together to transform disaster management and response in the coming decade.

An Afghan Media Tale

THOMAS FRESTON

When one thinks of Afghanistan the word "entrepreneurship" does not usually come to mind. More likely are such words as "war," "terrorism," "corruption," and "drugs." People tend to think of Afghanistan as a disaster zone, and in some places it still is. But there are also many areas of increasing prosperity and change and some key metrics that show great improvement. In some areas entrepreneurial activity has flourished and has probably done more to move the country forward with jobs, connectivity, and social change than anything else since the fall of the Taliban in 2001. In this chapter I will discuss the growth of communication and media as two of the biggest success stories in this war-torn nation.

Western countries' approach to Afghanistan has been primarily military-focused and very expensive. The United States alone spent over $120 billion on military efforts in Afghanistan in 2011, a mind-boggling rate of some $10 billion a month. Consider that this was in a country that in 2011 had only an estimated $15 billion gross domestic product. Indeed, there have been many positive and expensive infrastructure projects over the years: roads, wells, and schools, as well as great advances in health care. But military efforts prevail and the long-promised "civilian surge" has never really materialized. The military has run the show and the all-in cost is about $1 million per year per soldier.

Largely ignored by the international media have been the great successes of some of the homegrown efforts of Afghan entrepreneurs to build businesses. Although some of these efforts may have been jump-started with Western aid, in many cases they now operate profitably. The cell phone industry may be the greatest example. There are currently five cell phone companies operating in the country. In 2001, when the Taliban was in power, there were only 10,000 landlines in a country of 27 million people. There were a few satellite phones, but they were almost entirely in the hands of government officials and Al Qaeda. Afghanistan was not connected to the outside world at all, a common thread in its entire history. It has always been "off the grid," something that accounts for many of the conditions there.

In fact, forget the outside world—Afghans have never even been connected to *each other*. It has always been a rural, landlocked, mostly illiterate country cut-off from all sides. There has been a small urban elite, but no real media or communication infrastructure. Attempts to change this happened in the 1960s and 1970s, but the series of terrible events that began with the communist coup in 1978 put an end to that. Afghanistan gradually descended into chaos, first with the Soviet invasion, then the destructive civil war, all capped off with the ascent of the Taliban to power in 1996. All of this just further isolated the country. During the rule of the Taliban it was as if the country had moved back to the Middle Ages; a country on another planet.

Flash forward to 2012 and there are 17 million cell phones; over 60 percent of the country has them. Everywhere you go you see outdoor advertising for the various cellular operators, as well as the countless stores and stalls that sell them and the prepaid cards they require. This has had an immense impact on almost everything. People are connected to each other for the first time in their history. Farmers can find out the current price for produce that they want to bring to market. Businessmen can find out when the goods they have ordered might arrive. Families can reach each other, whether on the other side of town or the other side of the country. Women can find out if communal water taps are open and can access all types of information, including, for example, getting texts on prenatal care.

Banking services became available on cell phones as well. Realize that 97 percent of Afghans did not have bank accounts before the advent of cell phones and you can imagine how revolutionary this was.

Suddenly, many types of financial transactions could be performed on cell phones. The cell phone, entirely leapfrogging landline technology, has greatly improved the standard of living and economic conditions, led to the development of many kinds of new businesses, created many jobs, and opened the door to the more efficient modern world. Afghanistan needed infrastructure. Cell phone technology was the first piece to fall into place and the Afghans themselves performed this essential part of "nation building," albeit with some assistance from private foreign companies and foundations.

My own history with Afghanistan goes back to the early 1970s. As a young man I traveled there as part of a personal world tour, a sort of a "gap year" before that term existed. I had traveled overland from Europe through Turkey and Iran. I was immediately taken with the country. It was as far away as I had ever been and I loved it and felt strangely at home. The land was vivid, alive, and brutally beautiful. The people were hospitable and had a great sense of hospitality and dignity. Fascinated, I covered as much of the country as possible.

In those days Afghanistan was a very peaceful place, and had a peaceful Sufi vibe. Arianna Afghan Airlines, the national carrier, even had an advertising slogan: "Say Afghanistan and You Think of the World's Friendliest Country." Then it was entirely believable. Everyone I knew there would have agreed, but unfortunately now that's about the last phrase that would come to mind. Back then you would never worry about your personal security; you could walk alone anywhere. I spent days walking every back street in old Kabul, and even walked on the heads of the famed giant Buddhas of Bamiyan (blown up by the Taliban in 2001).

Entirely hooked, I decided to start a business there, as well as a parallel one in India, designing and making contemporary clothing, exporting it, and selling it to stores in North America and Europe. I had quick and surprising success. My main goal was to see if I could support myself living in Kabul and New Delhi, and indeed I did, spending some eight years in and out of those countries. It was the time of the birth of airfreight. The 747 had just arrived. One could make something in Kabul or Delhi and have it for sale in New York or London just a day later. It was also a fascinating time to live in Afghanistan as the people had a great yearning to connect to the modern world. This was what is now called Afghanistan's "Golden Age"—the 1960s and 1970s. Although still a conservative Muslim country, back then you might have spotted a woman in a miniskirt in Kabul. Change and progress were very much in the air.

All this came to an end for the Afghan people, and for me, with the "Saur Revolution" in April 1978, which brought a communist government to power, albeit one with very thin popular support. We later found out that this coup, which shocked the Afghans, was also met with surprise and skepticism by the Soviet Union. The Soviets invaded a year later to try and save the new regime from the popular unrest they had created. All this, as we know, led to decades of conflict and chaos, as well as one of the biggest refugee migrations in history. Millions died, millions more became refugees, the elite largely decamped to other countries, and the country's agricultural and educational capabilities, as well as much of the traditional tribal structure, were all but destroyed. A returnee now cannot help but note that the country is flooded with weapons, and that a much more austere form of Islam prevails. There is still considerable struggle and poverty, and the majority of Afghans have only known war in their lifetime. In 2011 it was ranked the third-poorest country in the world.

After a year in India I returned, saddened, to New York in 1980 and began a new career in the media and entertainment business. I got a job at a startup company that went on to develop MTV, Nickelodeon, Comedy Central, and many other specialized new "cable TV" channels. This was the "cable TV revolution," and I was on the front lines. This revolution worked out much better for me. I soon became the CEO of MTV Networks, then the CEO of its parent company, Viacom. We pioneered many businesses but I was most proud of, and involved with, our international activities. We were the leaders and innovators in this regard, creating many localized cable and satellite networks of our TV brands throughout the world. As the media world began to deregulate in Europe, South America and, finally, Asia, it was possible for private companies to enter the business. We were first movers.

In Asia we moved west from Hong Kong, starting networks as far as India, where I was able to witness firsthand the explosive growth of cable TV in that country. India had just begun its economic reforms and, with the Gulf War in 1991, there was an intense interest in CNN and their war coverage. Indian entrepreneurs set up satellite dishes and ran cables down the sides of streets. A new industry was born and it went on to become one of the most dynamic and remarkable TV markets in the world as many domestic and international players jockeyed for position.

India, long a sluggish and bureaucratic country, aggressively developed this vibrant new industry that would go on to create countless jobs, incredible wealth, and many other opportunities and related businesses. The monopoly of the state as the sole television provider had been broken. This growth of television supercharged the consumer economy and with it came broad-scale consumer advertising and many new retail outlets and systems. India would never be the same.

More interesting to me, though, was the social impact that cable and satellite television was having, especially on women and the poor—not just in the cities but also in the rural areas, where much of life had been unchanged for centuries. Television, one of the most powerful tools ever created, began to accelerate the rate of social change in Indian rural communities as had never been seen before.

This rich new array of television choices piped into India's remote villages was not just entertaining but also conveyed a vast amount of information, exposure to the outside world, and behavioral signals. Almost immediately people would notice changes in dress styles, in personal hygiene, and in language. Most popular television shows were produced in urban settings where lifestyles were quite different from rural areas. Soap operas became the most popular format. The characters in them tended to have better educations, smaller families, and, perhaps most significant, a level of gender equality that was much healthier and balanced.

Many research studies showed the huge impact television quickly had on women's status in India. They reported significant attitude and behavior shifts, such as increased autonomy, an ability to go out without permission, contraceptive use, a desire for a smaller family size, a much lower acceptance of spousal abuse, and a reduced preference for sons over daughters. Even more notable is that these changes began to manifest within the first year of cable introduction.

Other findings were that investments in children's education and health increased when women had a greater voice in the household and that television clearly improved their voice in a big way. School attendance, especially with younger children, was found to increase after the introduction of cable television. Even latrine building accelerated. A most telling sign of belief in the power of TV to accelerate positive change came in 2006 when India's Tamil Nadu government distributed free color TVs to poor families, claiming that "nowadays it's not just about entertainment, it is more, it informs about health and public awareness issues."

A few years after the Indian "television revolution," it spread to the Arab world, another area where a large population had long been held hostage to state monopolies of TV and radio. Propaganda was always the primary purpose of the media, as was the promotion of a "national identity" rather than a regional one. In 1996 Al Jazeera, a panregional twenty-four-hour news channel in Arabic, was launched. Qatar, a small, rich Arab state, saw satellite television as a way to extend their influence beyond its borders. Called "a seed in the desert," Al Jazeera was a real breakthrough in what became a vibrant cross-border satellite marketplace. With the slogan "The opinion and the counter-opinion," it represented the next step in the global march of satellite and cable television. A big surprise to Arab governments, it was an instant hit with viewers across the region with its uninhibited political discussions and opened windows to the rest of the region and the world. It confronted many other taboos as well. Finally, the Arab government media monopoly had been broken. Things would never be the same.

Following Al Jazeera, Lebanon quickly launched a group of satellite networks, such as Future TV and LBC. Many more followed: a host of religious channels, news channels, women-oriented channels, general entertainment channels, and more. A satellite dish in Cairo in 2012 can pick up more than 700 different Arabic and international free-to-air TV signals. The impact of these channels, as it was in India, has been huge. People have begun to look beyond their single country, becoming much more aware of international developments. There is also a growing sense of a wider "Arab community." One could also say that the Arabic language itself began to get a bit more homogenized as the listener, long used to Egyptian dialect from movies and music, had wider exposure to unfamiliar accents.

As in India, women's sense of empowerment also increased. Now, even in this corner of the world where women have been historically unrepresented—whether in parliament or in the workforce—television is a much more equal-opportunity sphere. Female news anchors and personalities became common sights. Educated women regularly spoke about social issues and other subjects. While the long-term question of women's empowerment has yet to unfold in the Arab world, there is no doubt of the huge impact satellite television has had on opinions and on social and governmental issues. Look no further than the so-called "Arab Spring" of 2011. Facebook and Twitter are commonly cited as catalysts for this region-wide revolt against the status quo. However, while they certainly played a key role, satellite TV was much more influential, as it is more widely received and viewed, and had pointed out problems in these countries for years.

With all this in mind, an interesting stage was set for Afghanistan after the fall of the Taliban government in late 2001. What would happen? Afghanistan, after all, had less media than perhaps any place on earth. Prior to the Taliban regime there was little television access and it was a government monopoly with limited distribution and impact. The government monopoly also controlled radio access.

The Taliban came to power in 1996. Just when Al Jazeera was launching its signal, the Taliban was banning both TV and radio (along with music, shaving, and kite flying, among other things). Televisions were to be destroyed, and those caught with them were subject to imprisonment or floggings. As the world moved into the twenty-first century, Afghanistan moved into the fourteenth. People actually buried their sets in the ground in order to save them.

In 2004, well after the Taliban's ouster, a new constitution was created for Afghanistan. One of the more valuable and interesting provisions was for "freedom of the press," on the condition that the content was not contrary to the laws of Islam. This opened the door for the creation of a truly independent media sector. The Western coalition saw an independent media as essential for the creation of a durable democracy. So did some Afghans. One such person, watching events unfold, was Saad Mohseni, an Afghan émigré who returned to the country in 2002. As Mohseni told CNBC in 2010 about returning, "back in 2002 there were so many of us coming back, full of optimism. We were looking for opportunities to invest money and it became evident that media was non-existent."

Mohseni is the CEO for the family company Moby Media—the nation's leading commercial media group. Moby consists of fifteen different media companies: radio and television stations, recording and production companies, publishing and advertising firms, and a small magazine. The portfolio includes the Farsi-language Tolo TV, the country's leading broadcaster, as well as Lemar TV, a companion Pashto language network, and Tolo News, a twenty-four-hour satellite news channel (although satellite and cable in Afghanistan is very limited). In addition, they program a transnational commercial satellite network, "Farsi1," that covers some 100 million Farsi speakers in Iran, the United Arab Emirates, and Uzbekistan, among other countries. It is a joint venture with News Corporation and is based in Dubai.

Many other entrepreneurs began commercially supported media companies as well. As of 2012 it was estimated that Afghanistan had some seventy-five different TV stations and over 200 radio stations. Kabul's electronic media environment quickly became as rich and diverse as many of the world's capital cities. In 2011 it had some thirty terrestrial television networks (only two state-run) and forty-two different radio stations.

Independent media, along with cell phones, has been the nation's biggest business successes. In spite of intermittent electricity and an initial lack of televisions, the business has exploded. Color televisions from China can be purchased for as little as $75 and they are omnipresent. You can see them everywhere: in the bazaars, in stores, and being lugged around to people's homes. Antennas can be seen sticking up in the most unlikely places. Sometimes televisions are connected to car batteries for power. Restaurants, teahouses, and other public places have them on prominent display, so impact and reach is considerable, particularly in urban areas. It was estimated in 2011 that about 55 percent of Afghans have direct access to television. Remember, Afghanistan was the third-poorest country in the world and, officially, had no television as recently as 2001.

As all this was happening I was in the tail end of my media career in New York City. But I had still been following events in Afghanistan from a safe distance ever since I left in 1978. It is a hard country to get out of your system and I was still enchanted by it. In 2005 I met a smart, adventurous young American woman of Iranian descent in New York City, Sarah Takesh. She had grown up in the United States but, fascinated with Afghanistan, had made her way there in 2002 after college and graduate school. She set up a clothing business, much as I had some thirty years earlier. I was eager to finally get a firsthand report about Afghanistan and the capital, Kabul. The city was open to the outside world again and I listened avidly as she recounted the scene in this newly liberated country, along with the trials and tribulations of running a clothing-for-export business there. We compared a lot of notes. When she left she said, "You must meet my boyfriend one day, Saad Mohseni. He runs a media company there and is considered 'sort of the Rupert Murdoch' of the country." About two months later I met Mohseni on a visit he made to New York City.

Mohseni was friendly, funny, and impeccably dressed. He is a charismatic man and seems to be in perpetual motion. It was clear that being a media mogul, in the home of the original moguls, is a relentless job. The challenges of building a modern business in a country that was still very much a disaster zone were considerable. There was no labor pool of trained television professionals. There was little to no electricity, little security, few existing advertisers, and, finally, no real consumer culture to speak of. Add to that the fact that this brand new independent media was under regular assault from various quarters. Television was still viewed suspiciously by many in power, and, to the most conservative members of the government, was seen as un-Islamic.

Despite all this Mohseni had become its most articulate champion. There had been arrests of Tolo TV news reporters after complaints from Afghan politicians, unaccustomed to media scrutiny, and demands that certain programming, such as an Indian soap opera, be taken down because it offended the country's conservative elite and glorified "idol worshipping." This became subject of one of Mohseni's many court cases. President Karzai once told Mohseni that he did not understand Afghan culture. Mohseni replied that "80 percent of Afghans with televisions have watched an Indian soap opera," and that this was one of the few forms of entertainment they had and could always change the channel if offended. Karzai said that the people are uneducated. Mohseni retorted, "You can't say they are mature enough to vote for you but not mature enough to change the channel." The soap opera stayed on the air, although with some digitized blurring of Hindu deities.

I stayed in touch with Mohseni and he would send me DVDs of some of his programming and keep me up to date. In turn, I introduced him to many in the U.S. media establishment. When I left Viacom in the fall of 2006 I accepted Mohseni's invitation to return to the country. Excited to finally return, I became quickly fascinated by the challenges and realities of this new Afghanistan. In time I became an advisor and board member of Moby Media.

At Moby I actually saw many similarities to my early days at MTV. Certainly not content-wise, but in the way it was staffed and the way it was programmed, produced, scheduled, and sold. At MTV we could not find any pool of television professionals that could produce at the low costs cable television then required. At both MTV and Moby we had to train ourselves and learn on the run. In both cases we hired young employees, people in their mid-to-late twenties. There was little money to produce programming, so, in the beginning, foreign programming was licensed and then dubbed. The first original programming was on the news and public information front.

Innovation and creativity prevailed there. The Moby offices and studios grew rapidly and soon became a warren of interconnected, repurposed residential buildings, all cobbled together on a well-fortified street filled with Kalashnikov-toting security guards. Visit the Moby offices and you got a sense as to what a new Afghanistan could look like. You'd see young, well-dressed Afghan men and women working side by side, collegially, politely, and energetically.

Mohseni and his competitors actually created the beginnings of a consumer culture in Afghanistan, something that never existed before.

The only advertising I remembered from thirty years ago were amusingly misspelled hand-lettered signs ("Weeding Cake Centar") and billboards reminding you about the death penalty for this or that transgression. Today billboards and advertising are everywhere and commercials for telephone service, banks, soft drinks, soaps, and shampoo are all over the TV and radio. New consumer products continue to be launched, backed by companies who want access to these previously untapped 30 million consumers.

Tolo TV has long been the market leader in Afghanistan: bold, innovative, and willing to invest in new original programming formats. Together with Lemar and Tolo News, it is estimated that the three channels hold over a 50 percent share of TV viewing in the country, a viewership that sharply skews to urban areas. They compete with religious channels, political channels, other general entertainment channels, and the state-run channels, but remain the industry leader. Tolo and Lemar run down-the-middle, populist fare; it's neither a propaganda outlet nor the Afghan version of Masterpiece Theater. They keep their finger on the pulse of the young country and are a conscious force for subtle, social change. Gender equality was put on top of their agenda. Tolo became a network where you'd see women read the news, or speak in a casual, friendly manner to men while cooking or during a call in the show. Just seeing a woman laugh on TV was revolutionary. They found early on, too, as in India, that television was inspirational. On Tolo people dressed well, shaved, and had nice homes and furniture. The general population became more conscious of this and followed suit.

In 2012 Tolo is producing some sixteen hours of original programming a day, an ambitious amount for any network. Much of this was news and information programming, which are among the most popular shows. "In Afghanistan you have to watch the news to survive; in the U.S. it's like a hobby," says Mohseni.

In 2011 Tolo launched a Farsi version of *Sesame Street* in coordination with Children's Television Workshop in the United States. It is a complete Afghanized version, produced in Kabul, and called *Baghch-e-Simsim*. It became an immediate success. Research studies showed that parents found it culturally appropriate, helpful in persuading fathers to allow their daughters to go to school, and it boosted children's enthusiasm for learning. Most viewers recommended it to others. Its positive impact was huge.

Tolo TV's biggest hit has been *Afghan Star*, a musical talent competition show much like *American Idol*, where contestants wage huge countrywide campaigns to win. It's estimated that over two-thirds of the country's population watches the finale episode, and the show gets more votes than the presidential election. It's such a hit that, when there are electricity shortages, the government doesn't turn off the electricity until the show is over. Music had been banned by the Taliban's regime, so its success is even more notable. It is creating a whole new generation of Afghan musical stars. Their story has resonated internationally as well; a documentary, *Afghan Star*, won an award at the 2009 Sundance Film Festival and was shown on HBO.

Moby and its competitors have challenged and confronted many people in power and they have plenty of critics among the politicians and the mullahs. In Afghanistan, no one had seen this sort of thing before. "Getting shut down, killing one of our people, bombing our facility, a staged riot, which is a favorite of people in our region—we fear all those things," Mohseni told me. But he still believes there's a degree of sophistication now about the media that didn't exist before. Politicians are more tolerant, and also increasingly aware of how to use the media effectively themselves. This is even true for the Taliban. Mohseni once received a call from a Taliban spokesman who had a bone to pick about the coverage of all the horrific things the Taliban was doing, such as planting improvised explosive devices and conducting suicide bombings. The spokesman didn't complain about too much coverage; he complained about too little.

The level of confidence in the media in Afghanistan is quite positive. While there are certainly some concerns about content, which is not unusual, they pale in comparison to what people see as its benefits. In a country where all three branches of government are seen to be insufficient and largely ineffective, the media, the "fourth estate," takes on a higher status than you would normally see in a developed country. Studies indicate that people view the media as their primary source of reliable information and as a positive societal force in general, regularly addressing issues of concern like crime, corruption, drugs, and the economy.

Something that did not exist before 2001 has assumed the amazing power to open minds and educate and become a watchdog over government, a promoter of national unity, and an effective way to keep up on the progress of the country's reconstruction. Lastly, on top of all this, it is a provider of entertainment. Afghans have very few entertainment choices; it is not like people can go out at night to dinner or a movie. The luxury of being entertained in your home is seen as a rare pleasure.

Despite all the corruption, misery, waste, and continued conflict, Afghanistan is in much better shape than it was in 2001. There has been substantial, yet fragile, progress in the first decade after the fall of the Taliban, and this progress should not be drowned out by the constant stream of bad news that we hear from the media. USAID data revealed in 2011 that life expectancy had risen from forty-five, once second-lowest in the world, to sixty-one. Infant mortality has been halved. Access to health care (within an hour) rose to 85 percent versus a mere 9 percent under the Taliban. In 2011 there were 10,000 schools against a mere 1,200 under the Taliban. By 2011 6.3 million children were in school, including 2.5 million girls. Not one girl was in school during the Taliban's time and, incidentally, these schools had seven times the number of teachers. The economy has grown rapidly. The country is also more urbanized, some 35 percent of the population, and the people, particularly young people, are more sophisticated than at any point in their history. War-related deaths are down considerably. According to the World Bank, in the 1990s about 9,000 people were killed a year.

We do not know how things will turn out in Afghanistan. The insurgency continues, the government struggles, and the international forces are preparing to depart by 2014, leaving behind mostly trainers for the Afghan National Army. That is a force of considerable size and, hopefully, it is one competent enough to protect the state and allow progress to continue. Optimists always point to one piece of data when accessing the prospects of Afghanistan resisting a new Taliban takeover once international forces are gone: survey after survey has concluded that two-thirds of the population consistently say they have "no sympathy for the Taliban."

However, two other issues, often unspoken, mitigate against this: the inadequacy of the current Afghan government, thought to be corrupt and predatory, and the continued support for the Taliban by Pakistan. In Pakistan the Taliban find not just sanctuary and funding, but also strategic support from at least some elements of the government. They want a pro-Pakistan, and anti-Indian, government in Kabul, and the Taliban fill that bill. Pakistan helped put the Taliban in power the last time around and was one of the three countries to diplomatically recognize them. Presumably they would like a similar outcome this time.

Perhaps there will be a political settlement with the Taliban and possibly they will accept the terms of the new Afghan constitution and live side by side with the rest of the population. It is hard to say. But one other factor works in Afghanistan's future, one that has only come about since 2001, and that is the fact that, while still physically landlocked, Afghanistan is now increasingly technologically unlocked to the outside world and its modern cultural, social, and economic forces. Like the Indians and the Arabs before them, Afghans finally have a window to the outside world and with that has come a slow tide of positive change, particularly among the large, new, educated urban generation. These young men and women are connected to each other and to the forces of modernity and globalization, via the internet, Facebook, increased education, improved English-language abilities, and, importantly, to the exposure of the multitude of private television channels.

Young urban Afghans increasingly see their future in the world outside, not in following the practices of the older generations who have kept the country in disaster mode for so long. Looming in their favor is the fact that Afghanistan is an extremely young country, the second-youngest in the world, with a median age of just seventeen. Incredibly, half of the population there is *under* seventeen. Maybe the old stereotypes and thinking that brought the country decades of war and misery can slowly be transformed as these people age out. The Afghans, especially the young ones, are not the same people they were in 2001. One trusts that the country will not turn back from this progress and revert to the past. As the saying goes, "There is too much toothpaste out of the tube. It won't go back."

It is a novel thought, but television and other media have emerged as a new and potentially effective tool for disaster relief under certain conditions. Its impact on social change, education, and health can easily be overlooked, but it is significant. Television is one of the most powerful instruments ever known to man for communicating ideas and providing a window to the world, so why not consciously try to utilize that power smartly when possible? In Afghanistan we have seen disaster mitigated to some extent in the last ten years by television and other media. It has managed to inform, build pride, create heroes, educate, connect people to each other and the outside world, and build a sense of community, identity, nationhood, and progress. Importantly, it has been able to do all of this through homegrown movements in spite of low levels of literacy and electricity and without a lot of outside funding. It has been one of Afghanistan's few success stories and one of the best uses of "soft power" we've ever seen.

Terror, Transformed

A Financier's Journey into Social Entrepreneurship

MICHAEL POLLACK

My story begins innocuously, with a dinner reservation in a world-class hotel. The first part of the story ends twelve hours later after the Indian Army freed us. The second part is, and will forever be, a work in progress: to give back, in the fullest way possible, to a nation that taught me the value of life and how beauty can exist in tragedy.

My point is not to sensationalize events. It is to express my gratitude and pay tribute to the staff of the Taj Mahal Hotel in Mumbai, whose actions and sacrifice in the face of disaster serve as an inspiration for my philanthropic activity.

On November 26, 2008, my wife Anjali and I along with another couple arrived at the Taj around 9:30 p.m. for dinner at the Golden Dragon, one of the better Chinese restaurants in Mumbai. We were a little early, and our table wasn't ready, so we walked next door to the Harbour Bar. We had barely begun to enjoy our beers when the host told us our table was ready. We decided to stay and finish our drinks.

Thirty seconds later, we heard what sounded like a heavy tray smashing to the ground. This was followed by twenty or thirty similar sounds and then absolute silence. We crouched behind a table just feet away from what we now knew were gunmen. Terrorists had stormed the lobby and were firing indiscriminately.

We tried to break the glass window in front of us with a chair, but it wouldn't budge. The Harbour Bar's hostess, who had remained at her post, motioned to us that it was safe to make a run for the stairwell.

She mentioned, in passing, that there was a dead body right outside in the corridor.

We made our way up the stairwell and took refuge in the small office of the kitchen of another restaurant, Wasabi, on the second floor. Its chef and staff served the four of us food and drink and even apologized for the inconvenience we were suffering.

Over the next two hours, through text messaging, e-mail on Black-Berrys, and a small TV in the office, we realized the full extent of the terrorist attack on Mumbai. We figured we were in a secure place for the moment. There was also no way out.

Outside the kitchen was abuzz as the staff sought to organize and secure the guests. Then, suddenly, the kitchen went dead silent. We instantly closed the office door, barricaded it with a large table, and turned off the lights. The four of us and one staff member crouched in silence. Within five minutes there were powerful, pounding knocks on the door. A man on the other side of the door shouted something in either Hindi or Urdu. We froze.

Twenty minutes of still silence passed as if it were days, then we heard soft tapping on our door: "It's OK to come out now. We have a safer place for you to hide," a gentle voice said in English.

We quietly debated, then gingerly emerged from the office. Greeting us with a wide smile was Vijay Banja, a prominent chef at the hotel. He led us down a hallway to an area of the Taj known as The Chambers. In there we met a few hundred other guests. The staff had spontaneously reacted, organizing hundreds of guests from all over the hotel and bringing them to what they felt was the safest, most secure area in the hotel.

Initially the mood inside The Chambers was calm, even cautiously optimistic. But then, a member of parliament phoned into a live TV newscast and let the world know that hundreds of people—including CEOs, foreigners, and members of parliament—were "secure and safe in The Chambers together." Adding to the escalating tension and chaos was the fact that, via text and cell phone, we knew that the dome of the Taj was on fire only a few floors above us.

As the mood became increasingly tense I called my wife's cousin, who was the guardian of our children, and told her what our wishes were for the children should we not survive. Vijay, seeing how nervous Anjali and I were, approached. "Don't worry," he said. "Be calm. If anything has to happen I'll die before you," he added gently.

"But I don't want you to die," Anjali responded, holding his hand.

It wasn't just an interested public that was listening to the TV broadcasts. The terrorists' handlers too were actively listening in Karachi. Through the use of satellite phones they informed their four mindless automatons to find and target The Chambers.

The staff didn't know about the satellite phones, but they did know they had a huge problem. They saw that the terrorists were now actively seeking The Chambers. They didn't have a choice; at around 2 a.m., they attempted an evacuation. We all lined up to head down a dark fire escape. But after five minutes, grenade blasts and automatic-weapon fire pierced the air. A mad stampede ensued to get out of the stairwell and take cover back inside The Chambers.

After that near-miss, Anjali and I decided we should hide in different rooms. While we hoped to be together at the end, our primary obligation was to our children. We wanted to keep one parent alive. Because I am American and she is Indian, and news reports said the terrorists were targeting U.S. and U.K. nationals, I believed I would further endanger her life if we were together in a hostage situation.

So when we ran back to The Chambers I hid in a toilet stall with a floor-to-ceiling door and she stayed with our friends, who fled to a large room across the hall.

For the next seven hours, I lay in the fetal position, keeping in touch with Anjali periodically via BlackBerry. I was joined in the stall by Joe, a Nigerian national with a U.S. green card. I managed to get in touch with the FBI, and several agents gave me status updates throughout the night.

Meanwhile, Anjali and the others were across the corridor in a mass of people lying on the floor and clinging to each other. People barely moved for seven hours, and for the last three hours they felt it was too unsafe to even text. While I was tucked behind a couple walls of marble and granite in my toilet stall, she was feet from bullets flying back and forth.

The ten minutes around 2:30 a.m. were the most frightening. We heard single, punctuated shots ring through the air. The terrorists were literally within feet of us, and hunting. We were separated by a thin door with a standard lock. The lights were off, and our lives hung in the balance. The Indian Army had yet to arrive. If the terrorists walked through that door we were dead. Everyone was in deep prayer and most, Anjali included, had accepted that their lives were likely over. It was terrorism in its purest form. No one was spared.

I cannot even begin to explain the level of adrenaline running through my system at this point. It was this hyper-aware state where every sound, every smell, every piece of information was ultra-acute, analyzed and processed so that we could make the best decisions and maximize the odds of survival.

Was the fire above us life-threatening? What floor was it on? Were the Indian Army commandos near us, or were they terrorists? Why is it so quiet? Did the commandos survive? If the terrorists come into the bathroom and to the door, when they fire in, how can I make my body as small as possible? If Joe gets killed before me in this situation, how can I throw his body on mine to barricade the door? If the Indian commandos liberate the rest in the other room, how will they know where I am? Do the terrorists have suicide vests? Will the roof stand? How can I make sure the FBI knows where Anjali and I are? When is it safe to stand up and attempt to urinate?

Eventually the terrorists realized their mistake and sought to go through the doors they had previously passed. To our good fortune, the Indian Army had arrived (around 4 a.m.) and tried to secure our position. The next five hours were filled with the alternating sounds of pin-drop still silence combined with sudden bursts of an intense, sporadic grenade/gun battle between the Indian commandos and the terrorists. It was fought in pitch-black darkness; each side was trying to outflank the other. The Indian Army lacked both night vision goggles and closed circuit communication equipment. They were also totally unfamiliar with the Taj, a sprawling century-old Mumbai landmark. Additionally, many in the army were armed with only single-shot, bolt action rifles, making the terrorists better armed with only AK-47s. The outcome was far from certain.

As I lay cowering on that bathroom floor, not knowing whether Anjali was still alive, or whether I would make it out alive myself, I did what any good hedge fund manager would do; I made a trade with God. If He allowed me to survive, I would find a way to give back and truly do something "good" in the world.

By the time dawn broke, the commandos had successfully secured our corridor. A young commando led out the people who had been packed into Anjali's room. A few minutes after Anjali had been evacuated, Joe and I peeked out of our stall. We saw multiple commandos and smiled widely. I had lost my right shoe while sprinting to the toilet so I grabbed a sheet from the floor, wrapped it around my foot and proceeded to walk over the debris to the hotel lobby.

The corridor was laced with broken glass and bullet casings. Every table was turned over or destroyed. The ceilings and walls were littered with hundreds of bullet holes. Bloodstains were everywhere, though, fortunately, there were no dead bodies to be seen.

Anjali and I embraced for the first time in seven hours in the Taj's ground floor entrance. I did not know whether she was dead or injured because we had not been able to text for the past three hours.

Thanks to the brave actions of the staff and later the commandos, the terrorists never made it into The Chambers that night. Sadly, though, many of the staff who had guided us to our hiding place were not as fortunate. We later learned that after locking the doors leading to The Chambers, many had remained on the other side of those doors, and several were killed (the same doors the terrorists had miraculously decided not to force their way through). They were the victims of the single shots we heard. Of the thirty-six people who died in the Taj that night, twelve were staff, including Vijay Banja.

Vijay lived three blocks away from the Taj and, having intimate knowledge of its layout, could have left at any point in time that night to return safely to his wife and son. No one would have faulted him had he left. But he, and the rest of the Taj staff, chose to stay. Hundreds of us are alive today thanks to their collective action. They made the ultimate sacrifice that night, a sacrifice I seek to feel worthy of every single day.

After

I returned to New York a few days later. My world was ablaze. I had experienced beauty in the face of disaster. The staff had felt it was their duty to protect and serve us, now it was my duty to fulfill the promise I made on that bathroom floor. "Charity given out of duty, without expectation of return, at the proper time and place, and to a worthy person is considered to be in the mode of goodness" (Bhagavad Gita 17.20).

I had spent the prior decade on Wall Street. In 2001, barely two years out of college, I had been in the right place at the right time with the right skill set. I partnered with a man sixteen years older than I, and together we started an investment firm in what then was a little-known niche industry, hedge funds. Unbeknownst to either of us at the time, we were to ride one of the greatest modern day waves of wealth creation. Over the eight years we worked together, industry assets grew from $300 billion to $2 trillion in 2008. Our returns were powerful and our firm's assets under management swelled from $50 million to $2.5 billion. I felt like one of Horatio Alger's heroes. It was a dream come true.

After the attacks, however, I realized that wealth is nothing in and of itself. It is just potential power; what matters is what you do with that power. So I resolved to make use of my wealth to do something worthwhile. Over the next month I dissolved my relationship with my business partner, and established a philanthropic foundation.

I named my foundation "SCA" or "Sat, Chit, Ananda" (which loosely translates as "existence, knowledge, bliss"). The phrase comes from the Upanishads (ancient Sanskrit texts) and, for me, embodies one of the great essences of humanity—that we exist for a speck of time, but have the ability to grow our knowledge base such that we can make better decisions in order to come closer to achieving our potential in life, and the fulfillment of that potential approximates "bliss."

Consciousness is our one major evolutionary advantage over the rest of the animal kingdom. With consciousness comes language and the ability to learn, refine, and improve our decisions. We know from science that raw intelligence is evenly distributed both geographically and across the socioeconomic strata. We also know from practical experience, and countless studies, that access to high-quality education is not evenly distributed. Therefore, I came to view the quality of, and access to, education as one of the great social missions of the twenty-first century.

The four young men who killed those thirty-six people at the Taj, and who would have killed us, came from poor areas in Pakistan. They were gullible cannon fodder; doped up zombies whose handlers were able to channel teen angst with aberrant religious interpretations in a complex geopolitical game they had hardly an inkling of, or ability to understand. Where would they have been if they were born and educated on the Upper East Side of Manhattan? Where is Pakistan now as a result of its religious *madrassas* and failed public educational system?

My point is not to excuse their actions. They are indefensible. It is to raise the question of the socializing influence of education and an educational system on youth. Plato likened education to putting "sight into blind eyes."[1] Birthplace greatly influences that sight. Will a child be "lucky" to enter a *madrassa* to become indoctrinated with dogma, or will he be empowered to pursue his life by developing critical analytic facilities learning how to read, write, and add?

Intent into Action

At my hedge fund I had spent my days analyzing companies and meeting with management teams in order to try to intelligently invest our partners' capital. Taking a parallel approach, my mission was now to find social entrepreneurs involved in education, help them develop their business models, and use my foundation's assets to help them expand the scope of their work.

I had never been to India for more than two weeks at a time. My experience was limited to major urban centers and tourist locations. I also had no idea of the nongovernmental organization (NGO) landscape. I had never supported an NGO outside of the United States, nor had I really done much business outside Mumbai.

Armed with a philosophical aim to find and support education-related NGOs, I poured myself into networking and learning about NGOs in India. The Indian NGO sector is rife with stories of fraud and corruption. In fact, most Indians, especially the older generation (like my father-in-law), regarded it with distrust. They are all too familiar with nepotism, payoffs, missing funds, and the like. As a result, a vast majority of all philanthropy in India goes to religious institutions. My foundation, which donates a few hundred thousand dollars per year, is actually considered "medium-sized" in India.

While India has 3.3 million NGOs,[2] there are only very few with multimillion dollar budgets that have institutional backing. In fact, there are only an estimated 500 that have budgets in excess of $100,000.[3] The vast majority are small, founder-led niche operations. I determined that I was going to target the NGOs with annual budgets of $150,000–$250,000 and see what I could do to help them scale to become institutional.

In order to help structure my search I decided to look for organizations that exhibited the following four criteria:

1. a high-energy, reputable social entrepreneur;

2. a cost-efficient, scalable business model serving a previously unmet need in the community;

3. strong operational and financial oversight; and

4. the use of local talent.

1. Leadership

Every organization, whether in government, the corporate world, or the not-for-profit world, succeeds or fails based upon the quality of its leadership. And no position is more important, particularly for not-for-profits, than the executive director. Unlike his or her peers in the corporate or government world, the executive director tends to exert a relatively greater degree of control on his or her organization in an NGO, particularly in the case of smaller, founder-led organizations.

Most executive directors are deeply empathic and have immense compassion for the cause they serve. This drive is what, by and large, sustains them through the long hours, poor pay, and initial rejection that accompany any new venture. They are fighters who have found and created a unique service or operating methodology that has enabled them to survive.

Where most executive directors fail, or at least fail in terms of achieving their potential scale, is when it comes to strategic planning. That is, he or she is so committed to his or her cause that they are blinded to certain realities of the marketplace. Achieving the right mix of pragmatism and idealism is an art, but without some level of pragmatism long-term viability and scale are impossible. As a result, it is important to have an executive director with both "head" and "heart."

2. Scalability, Measurability

Unfortunately, we live in a world of finite resources. This, combined with the premise that "all life is created equal" (which arguably is one of the guiding tenets of philanthropy), means difficult decisions must be made to prioritize and allocate resources.

It is a complex, imprecise, and often "unfair" process to attempt to quantify results. Since Jeremy Bentham presented the idea of utility in the eighteenth century, people have debated its measurability. Every field can only have precision to the extent allowable by that field in question. In mathematics we can have beautiful equations with definitive, absolute answers. Conversely, though, in social work, or anything human-related for that matter, we cannot expect exact precision. However, just because exact precision is not available does not mean that there cannot be reasonable yardsticks that can be used to attempt to qualify the success or failure of an organization.

Every organization must have a business plan. That business plan, whether it is a narrative written in prose or an Excel spreadsheet with numbers and categories, is benchmarked by measurable outcomes (children fed, vaccinations given, etc.). It states projections of what an organization hopes to accomplish given the best estimation of its present-day realities; the further out in time, the less likely the projections are to be accurate.

As the only constant in the world is change, no business plan will ever prove to be exactly right. That said, just because a business plan is never going to be completely accurate does not mean it cannot be measured. It is these measurable outcomes—agreed to in advance by funders and entrepreneurs alike—that serve as guideposts to whether an organization is achieving or failing in its mission.

When evaluating business plans prior to funding, one key metric has to be scalability; the capacity to ultimately reach and serve as many individuals as possible. If an organization can achieve its milestones and prove its mission statement, it will likely have the ability to attract additional resources to further its growth.

To put it into financial terms, looking for scalability is like getting a free call option. If you have two organizations that can both educate 1,000 children for the same cost, but one has the ability to grow to serve 100,000 while the other does not, it is clearly better to back the one that can achieve greater scale.

3. Strong Oversight

Perhaps the biggest impediment to the success of an NGO is corruption; ensuring that its funds are going where they are supposed to and that an organization is serving the people it is supposed to serve is paramount. The cardinal sin in philanthropy is misallocation of resources. Nothing can kill a promising organization quicker than the perception, or actualities of, improprieties.

The best possible oversight would be to have direct access to, and oversight of, the bank balances where funds are deposited and operating expenses are paid, although this is highly time-consuming for both the organization and the donor. The next best alternative, and prerequisite to funding any organization (except in acute disaster scenarios where it would take too long and result in an unacceptable human cost), are audited financials. Just about every country has government ministries and a system for accounting for the inflow and outflow of funds, and most require an audit in order for an organization to be eligible to receive foreign funds.

If direct access to bank balances and expenses is not available, and no credible audited financials exist, then directly serving on the organization's board, or at the very least having a close relationship with someone serving on the board, is necessary. Most of the time it is possible to get some independent third-party verification of results, which allows for some supervision over the utilization of funds.

4. Use of Local Talent

One of the great failures of Western-oriented philanthropy is the implicit or explicit intellectual imperialism of the donor. It is a sad fact that the golden rule of philanthropy is "he who has the gold rules." Failure often results from a lack of understanding of a population's needs, as they need them, through their own prism of life, and not through the donor's idealized norms.

Along those lines, in order to achieve sustainability an organization must be able to employ, train, and empower members of the local community. As the phrase goes, "give a man a fish and he'll eat for a day, teach him how to fish and he'll eat for a lifetime." The goal of NGOs is to impart knowledge and build competencies within the local populace, not to make recipients dependent on handouts.

Intellectual Abstraction Meets Reality

I had developed an abstract, intellectual framework. That was the easy part. Now I needed to apply it to real-life situations. After compiling a short list of potential NGOs I was interested in backing, I made it a point to visit each and every one of them in the field prior to funding. Fortunately, I had a lot of time, and an intense desire to see more of India, so in 2009 I spent three months there, visiting over forty NGOs in all parts of the country.

I never had a full appreciation for the diversity within India until I began to see it firsthand. India is more a subcontinent than it is a monolithic country; that is not to say that the country is not united around cricket, Bollywood, and a common currency, only that the difference in food, language, religion, and terrain is immense.

My father spent his career as a teacher in the California public school system, and my mother spent hers as a not-for-profit health-care executive. In high school and college I had volunteered as a tutor or teacher's aide in urban, low-income neighborhoods in the United States. After I graduated and became a working professional, I became philanthropically engaged at a board level in two different education-related organizations helping to improve New York City schools for those less fortunate. None of my work in the United States could prepare me for my experiences in India.

In Ahmednagar, a town 200 miles east of Mumbai, I visited an organization called CSW Help. CSW Help was run by Dr. G, a kind, warmhearted man in his fifties (names in this section only have been changed to protect anonymity). Dr. G was a professor at a local university who had been working with commercial sex workers (CSWs) and their children for over twenty years.

He was drawn to the plight of these women and their children while still a graduate student in college. The quintessence of charity is to attempt to empower those at the bottom of society, and it is hard to get much lower, especially in India, than CSWs, or their children.

The majority of CSWs are women from other states within India or abroad who have been sold into the profession by their families. They are pariahs within the cities they live, generally confined to the three blocks of the red light district that serves both as their "home" and their place of work. Routinely beaten, often substance abusers, they serve a clientele of truck drivers and military conscripts that pay them $0.75–$1.50 per "meeting" (the price depends on their age and attractiveness).

Even worse off than these women are their children. Oftentimes seen by their mothers as a nuisance who get in the way of work, they too are shunned by their communities and have no place to spend at night while their mothers work.

Dr. G started by first setting up night schools to teach these children, and later expanded to establish a residential facility, a medical facility for HIV positive patients, and even an orphanage. Dr. G had since grown CSW Help to support over 400 homeless destitute children in residential homes, provided shelter and vocational training to more than sixty women in distress, educated over 900 children in their slums, and was empowering and rehabilitating over 2,100 commercial sex workers to lead a better life.

With an annual budget of approximately $200,000, a well-respected executive director, substantial operating history, and fulfillment of a clear need in the community, I thought CSW Help the perfect type of organization to support, so I made the drive out to Ahmednagar to spend a few days with Dr. G in the field.

On our first day, Dr. G took me to a red light district where CSW Help works. The 100-square-foot "apartments" with bowed beds, drooping ceilings, stained linens, and dirty floors where these women worked and lived was scarring. Women in their thirties looked fifty. Their eyes were recessed, empty of life. Resigned to their fate, their heads hung devoid of energy. Dr. G told me he had been working in this red light district for fifteen years, and that not one of the original women he worked with was still alive. The majority had died of HIV/AIDS. He told me that the infection rate was more than 90 percent ten years ago, but now down to 30 percent as a result of his work.

Later, Dr. G took me to a different town, another red light district where he worked, except this one was different. CSW Help had built a community center in the heart of the red light district. Sitting in the hall of the new center the women told me the story of a truck driver who used to get drunk and beat one of the girls regularly. One night when he arrived, drunk and ready for assault, the women were prepared. As he attempted to beat one of them ten others came to her defense. The eleven women wound up beating this man so severely he had to be taken to the hospital and hasn't come back since.

These women, while forced into lives they would never want their children to lead, had a sense of agency and community, a sense that they were not just purely victims. They knew about disease prevention, and had banded together to force their clients to use condoms. Some of them were also receiving skills training in other professions and were looking to leave the CSW industry altogether. It was not a great life in the absolute sense, but it was definitely a better life than before.

Over the years, Dr. G had raised enough money from donors to establish a residential facility for the children of CSWs. He even had a separate wing for those women and their children who were born HIV positive. His was one of the first HIV outreach programs in India. On my visit I stayed at the facility close to the kids. It looked like any other boarding school; kids were excitedly playing cricket on the fields, the little ones sliding and climbing in the playground. Previously abandoned, marginalized children now had their own sense of community—a place where their background was irrelevant. The focus was on their future.

At the end of the visit, I was so moved by the warmth of Dr. G and the plight of the CSWs and their children that I made a grant on the spot towards improving the education of the children and the outreach/training of the CSWs.

More than just money, though, I wanted to help Dr. G improve his education outcomes, expand the scope of his work, and develop the infrastructure that would allow him to scale into institutional grants. Through my network I managed to find one of the world's leading academic researchers on female adolescents. She was a tenured, non-Indian Ivy League professor who had previously won a Fulbright to work with a similar, but significantly larger organization in South Asia. As it so happened she also was looking for a new project, and within a few months of reaching out to her, she and her assistant made the trip and were in Ahmednagar to assist CSW Help and meet Dr. G.

Her trip started in a manner familiar to many foreigners, a nice intestinal parasite that makes long car rides severely less enjoyable. That omen continued. When she arrived at CSW Help, Dr. G was nowhere to be found. After two days of travel, Dr. G was three hours late to their first meeting.

Unfazed, she proceeded to spend two weeks with CSW Help, and her assistant stayed an additional four weeks. One month after he returned they presented to CSW Help the outline of a comprehensive plan to measure educational outcomes, streamline organizational infrastructure, and grow CSW Help substantially.

I could not be more excited. My goal of trying to help Indian NGOs scale was now in full swing. However, there was one problem—Dr. G and CSW Help did not read the report, and in fact, did not even bother to acknowledge receipt of the report. In fact, they were not excited enough to even return phone calls from the experts who had volunteered their time. There was not even a real discussion.

I had failed to realize the political intricacies of Dr. G and his staff. They were not open to a true discussion. The organization was too political, with certain individuals having too much to lose with any substantial change. It wasn't that anyone was "bad" or "good," just that there was an inertia and comfort to their operations without a true desire inside of CSW Help to change anything. If the children in the CSW Help school were not learning to read and write in line with their peers, they were still in a place far better than they would be in without help. That was simply enough. If they did not want to implement objective, results-based education measurement procedures to grow their donor base, so be it. They had a local donor base that could support its operations, even if they had to shrink a little.

Three years later, CSW Help was still struggling to raise money to support its budget, serving roughly the same numbers of women and children, and still mired in the same internal political issues. As my resources are finite, and I, by necessity, must seek the highest and best use for them, I sadly discontinued my support of Dr. G and CSW Help. I had seen in CSW Help a vision of the future I wanted for them, not necessarily one that they wanted for themselves, nor one that they had the resolve to implement. In short, I looked to impose help where perhaps it was not needed. Lesson learned.

"Through Struggle Enlightenment"

A few months before I went to visit Dr. G I had met with another, equally remarkable, social entrepreneur, Safeena Husain. Safeena was the executive director of Educate Girls (EG). Working in Rajasthan, EG was a community organization and empowerment model that trained social workers to help rural, largely illiterate populations improve their

K-5 primary schools. They conducted teacher training, organized school management committees, and assisted local communities in the requisition of government funds. Importantly, EG also brought to schools their own curriculum for girl individuation; a curriculum that sought to turn girls from actors into agents, allowing them to ask questions as basic as "What do I want to be when I grow up?" (Rajasthan's historical legacy of sati [forced female self-immolation upon the death of a husband] speaks volumes to the gender gap in education that EG was trying to close.)

On one of my visits I met a ten-year old girl from a tribal village. Her family had thought her work too important to sacrifice so they had denied her the ability to go to school. Working with social worker from EG, she made a deal with her mother that she could go to school after she finished her work: she woke up every day at 5 a.m. to haul her firewood to market, then attended school. I will never forget how her eyes widened and how her face shone with excitement as she talked about learning to read, write, and add.

One of the great paradoxes of India is that it produces the largest number of college graduates in the world, yet is home to one-third of all acute poverty in the world. In Rajasthan, for example, only 15 percent of all school children can read a simple story in Hindi.[4] At the same time, there are so many well-educated college graduates in Rajasthan that the average starting salary of a social worker is only $1,500 per annum.

The power of the EG's model lies within its ability to train its social workers comprehensively and quickly, enabling each social worker to work in ten villages, or about twenty schools. With a staff of only twenty-five social workers EG was able to reach over 500 schools (about 70,000 children) at a cost of a mere $2 per child per year.

EG also had the ability and desire to scale; when I met Safeena they had just signed a memorandum of understanding with the state government in Rajasthan to cover the entire Pali district's 2,500 schools (reaching over 250,000 children). Additionally, the neighboring district of Jalore, after seeing the progress made in the pilot program in Pali, had reached out to EG to see if it could assist in its 2,000 schools (300,000 children).

The potential for EG to bring meaningful social change was clearly immense. Safeena had been hired and received funding to build out the initial pilot program of fifty schools in 2005. Within two years, she had validated the pilot and received more funds to help 500 schools, and now she was now on the cusp of scaling up to serve the full 2,500 schools in Pali.

The organizational challenge in front of Safeena was daunting. A Delhi-born, thirty-seven-year-old Muslim she was a graduate of the London School of Economics who had initially begun her career in Northern California working for a startup technology company. Finding that life unfulfilling she chose instead to take a low-paying position with an NGO aimed at helping the thirty-two Shuar tribes in the Ecuadorean Amazon jungle and working with communities in Mexico, Bolivia, and South Africa. Later she joined an Indian organization, spending two years in a rural town setting up a village school and rural clinic.

Safeena was a career NGO executive who had tremendous experience not only in management, but also—and this is equally as important—in direct fieldwork. On one of my visits I asked her why she did what she did and she gave me an answer I will never forget. She said, "Working in this little, little village in India I realized that we only get this one little life to live. So I began to ask myself what was I going to do with it to give it meaning? And in my work I find more meaning than I ever could in Silicon Valley."

The life of an executive director at an NGO like EG can be an isolating, stressful one, and Safeena is not immune to those pressures. In the field she is an outsider—an urban implant who dresses more Western than local and who speaks only Hindi, not the local dialect of Marwari. In Mumbai, where trips outside of urban centers are rare for the well-heeled, few can truly relate to the struggles of trying to grow and run an organization within the local bureaucratic system of Rajasthan. Add to that the pressures of running a donations-reliant organization that regularly only has a few months of cash on hand to fund its operations, and it is easy to see the stress of her position.

While I was extremely impressed with Safeena, I probably would not have supported her if it were just she alone attempting to scale and run EG. Safeena had partnered with Dasra, a McKinsey-like NGO consulting firm who introduced me to her initially. Founded by Neera Nundy and Deval Sanghavi, an equally energetic husband and wife team in their mid-thirties, Dasra had the ability to help Safeena grow her organization. Neera had been persuaded by Deval, a former Morgan Stanley banker himself, to ditch her pursuit of a corporate job after her Harvard MBA and instead move to Mumbai to start Dasra. Dasra had worked with a handful of other, highly successful, NGOs across India, and helped them achieve scale and move toward sustainability.

I run SCA in much the same way that I run my investment firm: by taking calculated risks. On the positive side, EG had world-class management, a scalable model, strong oversight, and employed local talent. On the negative side, it did not have the ability to measure results, nor adequate infrastructure to achieve its growth. EG was high-risk, but also potentially high-reward. Ultimately, though, in my estimation, the potential outweighed the risks and, with Dasra's backing, a friend and I, along with a wealthy Indian family, decided to fund the expansion of EG's work.

Over the next four years, I made numerous trips to rural Rajasthan to see EG's work in action, had monthly conference calls to review key budget and operational items, and attempted to use my network to fill in the pieces EG needed.

Crucially, as with CSW Help, I was able to use my Rolodex to provide an important piece of the puzzle: measurability. I introduced EG to researchers at Harvard and the University of Michigan, who agreed to help design a study, analyze outcomes, and report on results. Unlike CSW Help, however, Safeena, Dasra, and I were on the same page in terms of a business plan and model. I was also able to help link EG with a wonderful organization in Washington, DC, called Global Giving, which helped EG target smaller donors and now forms a meaningful part of their donor base.

Four years later, it worked. Initial data showed a doubling in Hindi literacy and a tripling of math skills pre- and post-EG services. The organization went from a skeleton infrastructure to having real depth. As a result, EG won numerous awards, and attracted multiple grants from institutional donors. EG's budget now exceeds $1 million and it now serves 500,000 children in India, making it one of the top NGOs in the country in terms of people served.

Conclusion

> Everything is quiet, peaceful, and against it all there is only the silent protest of statistics; so many go mad, so many gallons are drunk, so many children die of starvation. . . . And such a state of things is obviously what we want; apparently a happy man only feels so because the unhappy bear their burden in silence, but for which happiness would be impossible. It is a general hypnosis. Every happy man should have someone with a little hammer at his door to knock and remind him that there are unhappy people, and that, however happy he may be, life will sooner or later show its claws, and some misfortune will befall him—illness, poverty, loss, and then no one will see or hear him, just as he now neither sees nor hears others.[5]

The above is taken from the short story "Gooseberries" by the Russian physician and writer Anton Chekhov, *Gooseberries* (1898).

Anton Chekhov (1860–1904) was a physician who wrote at the dawn of industrialization when power was concentrated, the majority of people suffered, and information was scarcely distributed. Today, we live in the age of information. The "hammer" is omnipresent. Never before have so many been able to see, hear, and experience the lives of so many others so quickly. The Arab Spring of 2011, the tsunamis of 2006 and 2011, and the Haitian earthquake of 2010 were all dramatically brought into our homes through TV, Twitter, Facebook, and other forms of media.

The access to information brings upon us an imperative for action. However, while information is vastly more distributed, we are as constrained as ever in terms of resources and time. For these reasons I propose NGOs and donors consider the following four factors when looking to allocate resources: 1) a high-energy, reputable social entrepreneur;

2) a cost-efficient, scalable business model serving a previously unmet need in the community; 3) strong operational and financial oversight; and 4) the use of local talent.

The night of November 26, 2008, forever changed my life. I was given the gift, by strangers and by fate, to watch my children grow and develop. I was also given perspective on value. I believe that everyone in their own way seeks to give their life meaning, and while that quest may be universal, the answer to it is deeply subjective and personal. Anjali and I now know how lucky we are to be alive; how precious and fleeting life is; and how its ending is often arbitrary and unfair. We are also acutely aware of those who still suffer. We have tried our best to own, acknowledge, and channel this pain into something constructive—the education of children. For whatever we have given philanthropically in terms of time and resources, we have received far more back, and are forever thankful of that gift.

Introduction / Kevin M. Cahill, M.D.

1. Organisation for Economic Co-operation and Development (OECD), *Development: Aid to Developing Countries Falls because of Global Recession* (Paris: OECD, 2012).

Globalization, Growth, Poverty, Governance, and Humanitarian Assistance / Dominick Salvatore

1. The thirteen high-growth countries and the period of their high growth are: Botswana (1960–2005) Brazil (1950–80), China (1961–2005), Hong Kong, SAR (1960–97), Indonesia (1966–97), Japan (1950–83), Korea (1960–2001), Malaysia (1967–77), Malta (1963–94), Oman (1960–99), Singapore (1967–2002), Taiwan (China) 1965–2002, and Thailand (1960–97).

WFP: Organizational Maintenance in Uncertain Times / Masood Hyder

Disclaimer: Views expressed in this chapter are those of the author alone.

1. James T. Morris, "Africa's Food Crises as a Threat to Peace and Security," Statement of the Executive Director of the WFP to the UN Security Council, June 30, 2005.

2. Henk-Jan Brinkman, *World Food Programme: Fighting Hunger with an Updated Toolbox* (Rome: WFP, February 2010).

3. Henk-Jan Brinkman and Masood Hyder, "The Diplomacy of Specialized Agencies: High Food Prices and the World Food Program," in James P. Muldoon et al. (eds.), *The Dynamics of Multilateralism* (Boulder, CO: Westview Press, 2011).

4. UN Department of Safety and Security, communications to the author, February 2007 and March 2012.

5. According to the OECD, between 2002 and 2005 USAID's share of ODA decreased from 50 to 39 percent, while the share of the U.S. Department of Defense's increased from 6 to 22 percent. For further details see Paul Fishstein and Andrew Wilder, *Winning Hearts and Minds? Examining the Relationship between Aid and Security in Afghanistan* (Medford, MA: Feinstein International Center, Tufts University, January 2012).

6. OCHA 2011 *Humanitarian Appeal*, www.humanitarianappeal.net.

7. Brinkman and Hyder, "The Diplomacy of Specialized Agencies."

8. Development Initiatives website: www.globalhumanitarianassistance.org.

9. For studies on the future of the humanitarian enterprise, see works by Antonio Donnini of the Feinstein Institute, Tufts University.

10. James Q. Wilson, *Political Organizations* (Princeton: Princeton University Press), 1995.

11. Indian Embassy communication to WFP Country Director, Sudan, September 25, 2001.

12. WFP Executive Board, Annual Session, Rome, May 28–30, 2003.

13. *The Economist*, August 13, 2011, p. 13.

14. Author's interviews with staff of UN ExCom agencies in Beijing, Geneva, Jakarta, New York, Rome, and Washington, DC, 2004–7.

15. *Encyclopedia of Islam*, vol. 8 (1995) and vol. 11 (2002).

16. Jon B. Alterman with Shireen Hunter and Ann L. Phillips, *The Idea and Practice of Philanthropy in the Muslim World*, PPC Issue Paper No. 5, Bureau of Policy and Program Coordination, Muslim World Series (USAID: Washington, DC, September 2005).

17. Alex de Waal, "Towards a Comparative Political Ethnography of Disaster Prevention," *Journal of International Affairs* 59: 129–50.

18. Jeffrey D. Sachs, *The End of Poverty: Economic Possibilities for Our Time* (New York: The Penguin Press, 2005).

19. The arguments in this section concerning the threat posed by the hungry were originally presented by the author in "Humanitarianism and the Muslim World," *Journal of Humanitarian Assistance* (August 22, 2007).

20. Morris, "Africa's Food Crises." See also Olusegun Obasanjo, "Poverty's Handmaiden," *Guardian*, June 23, 2005 and his op-ed in *Toronto Star*, July 20, 2005.

21. Josette Sheeran, "How to End Hunger," *Washington Quarterly*, April 2010.

22. The Secretary-General's High-Level Task Force on the Global Food Crisis, *Comprehensive Framework for Action* (New York: United Nations, 2008).

23. E.H. Carr, *The Twenty Years' Crisis* (London: Macmillan, 1962), 93.

24. "Briefing: Africa's Hopeful Economies," *The Economist*, December 3, 2011.

25. Larry Minear, *The Humanitarian Enterprise* (West Hartford, CT: Kumarian Press, 2002), 209.

Disasters—A Nation's Experience in an Economic Recession / Ronan Murphy

1. The Organization for Economic Co-operation and Development (OECD) Development Assistance Committee, *Mid-Term Review of Ireland* (Paris: OECD, October 2011), 88.

2. Government of Ireland (GoI), *Irish Aid Annual Report 2010* (Dublin: GoI), 4.

3. Statement by Ireland's head of delegation at Donor Conference on the Reconstruction of Iraq, October 2003.

4. See Chris Flood, *The Tsunami: Ireland and the Recovery Effort, Final Report* (Dublin: Department of Foreign Affairs); GoI, *Irish Aid's Support to Tsunami Affected Countries: A Value for Money Review* (Dublin: GoI, 2006); Tsunami Evaluation Coalition (TEC), *Joint Evaluation of the International Humanitarian Response to the Indian Ocean Tsunami* (London: TEC, January 2007).

5. GoI, *White Paper on Irish Aid* (Dublin: GoI, 2006).

6. GoI, *Humanitarian Relief Policy* (Dublin: GoI, May 2009).

7. Mick Jackson of the Emergency Civilian Action Team briefed me on the security aspects of the visit.

8. Helen O'Neill, "Ireland's Foreign Aid in 2010," *Irish Studies in International Affairs* 22 (2011): 187–223.

9. I am grateful to Brendan Rogers and his colleagues in Irish Aid, especially David Bruck, for their help and comments. The views expressed are mine, as are any errors that may have been made.

What Can Modern Society Learn from Indigenous Resiliency? / Margareta Wahlstrom

1. National Information Center of Earthquake Engineering of India, *Guidelines for Earthquake Resistant Non-Engineered Construction* (Kanpur: Indian Institute of Technology, 2004). Available at www.traditional-is-modern.net/LIBRARY/GUIDELINES/1986IAEE-Non-EngBldgs/1986GuidelinesNon-Eng(ALL).pdf.

Providing for the Most Vulnerable in the Twenty-First Century / Flavia Bustreo, M.D.

This chapter draws from Dr. Bustreo's Distinguished Dean Guest Lecture at the Harvard School of Public Health in March 2011.

1. The Beijing Agenda for Global Action on Gender-Sensitive Disaster Risk Reduction, also known as the Beijing Declaration for Action, is a set of nine achievable actions before 2015 to ensure that a gender perspective is integrated into policies and

programs on disaster risk reduction and climate change adaptation. This plan of action was endorsed by participants from fifty countries, UN agencies and Civil Societies at the International Conference on Gender and Disaster Risk Reduction held at Beijing from April 20–22, 2009.

2. UNICEF, *Humanitarian Action for Children 2012* (Geneva: UNICEF, 2012).

3. WHO, *Make Every Mother and Child Count* (Geneva: WHO, 2005).

4. UNICEF, *Levels and Trends in Child Mortality* (Geneva: UNICEF, 2011).

5. WHO, *Gender and Health in Disasters* (Geneva: WHO, 2002).

6. UNICEF, *Humanitarian Action for Children.*

7. UNICEF, *The State of the World's Children* (Geneva: UNICEF, 1996), available at www.unicef.org/sowc96/contents.htm.

8. Family Care International, *Safe Motherhood: A Review* (New York: Family Care International, 2007), available at www.familycareintl.org/UserFiles/File/SM_A%20Review_Exec_Sum_%20FINAL.pdf.

9. UN, "Millennium Development Goals" (New York: UN, 2000), available at www.un.org/millenniumgoals/.

10. WHO, *Make Every Mother and Child Count.*

11. See the PMNCH website: www.who.int/pmnch/about/en/.

12. The G8 is an alliance of eight nations that convene at a yearly summit meeting to discuss global issues of political and economic importance. The members are France, the United States, the United Kingdom, Russia, Germany, Japan, Italy, and Canada. For more information visit the University of Toronto's G8 Information Centre (www.g8.utoronto.ca).

13. UNICEF, *The G8 Muskoka Initiative: Maternal, Newborn and Under-Five Child Health* (Geneva: UNICEF, 2010), available at www.unicef.org/media/media_54074.html.

14. African Union, *Assembly of the Union, Fifteenth Ordinary Session 25–27 July 2010, Kampala, Uganda,* available at www.africa-union.org/root/ua/Conferences/2010/juillet/Summit_2010_b/doc/DECISIONS/Assembly%20AU%20Dec%20289-330%20(XV)%20_E.pdf.

15. PMNCH, *Global Strategy for Women's and Children's Health* (Geneva: WHO, 2010), available at www.who.int/pmnch/topics/maternal/201009_globalstrategy_wch/en/index.html.

16. F. Bustreo et al., *Improving Child Health in Post Conflict Countries: Can the World Bank Contribute?* (Washington, DC: World Bank, 2005).

17. Ibid.

18. Ibid.

19. Ibid.

20. AMREF UK, "Achieving MDG 6 Will Require Considerable Investments in Human Resources for Health at All Levels," available at http://uk.amref.org/silo/files/achieving-mdg-6-will-require-considerable-investments-in-human-resources-for-health-at-all-levels.pdf.

21. WHO, *Reducing Child Mortality: The Challenges in Africa* (Geneva: WHO, 2007), available at www.who.int/pmnch/topics/mdgs/2008unchronicle_shoo.pdf.

22. WHO, *Global Shortage of Health Workers and Its Impact* (Geneva: WHO, 2006).

23. Vincent De Brouwere and Wim Van Lerberghe, *Safe Motherhood Strategies: A Review of the Evidence*, Studies in Health Services Organisation and Policy 17 (2001), available at http://seriousgiving.org/files/DWDA%202009/Interventions/Maternal%20Mortality/SafeMotherhoodStrategies.pdf#page=15.

24. Ibid.

25. F. Bustreo et al., *Improving Child Health in Post Conflict Countries*, 12.

26. UNICEF, *Paris Principles: The Principles and Guidelines on Children Associated with Armed Forces or Armed Groups* (Geneva: UNICEF, February 2007), available at www.un.org/children/conflict/_documents/parisprinciples/ParisPrinciples_EN.pdf.

27. The Global Fund, *Mid-Term Review of the Second Voluntary Replenishment 2008–2010, Cáceres, Spain, 30 March–1 April 2009: Progress Report on Aid Effectiveness*.

28. International Labour Organization, "C183 Maternity Protection Convention, 2000," available at www.ilo.org/ilolex/cgi-lex/convde.pl?C183.

Noncommunicable Diseases and the New Global Health / Thomas J. Bollyky

This chapter is adapted with permission from the author's article "Developing Symptoms," which appeared in the May/June 2012 issue of *Foreign Affairs*, vol. 91, no. 3.

1. World Economic Forum (WEF), *Global Risks 2009: A Global Risk Network Report* (Cologne/Geneva: WEF, 2009), 1, available at https://members.weforum.org/pdf/globalrisk/2009.pdf.

2. World Health Organization (WHO), *Global Burden of Disease Report* (Geneva: WHO, 1996), 1, 14, 16–17.

3. Rachel A. Nugent and Andrea B. Feigl, *Where Have All the Donors Gone? Scarce Donor Funding for Non-Communicable Diseases*, Center for Global Development Working Paper 228 (2010), 17.

4. WHO, *Scaling up Action against Noncommunicable Diseases: How Much Will It Cost?* (Geneva: WHO, 2011), 5.

5. Toni Johnson, "Global Action on Non-Communicable Diseases," Council on Foreign Relations (CFR) Backgrounder, September 21, 2011, available at www.cfr.org/health-and-disease/global-action-non-communicable-diseases/p25826.

6. Sheri Fink and Rebecca Rabinowitz, "The UN's Battle with NCDs," *Foreign Affairs*, September 20, 2011, available at www.foreignaffairs.com/articles/68280/sheri-fink-and-rebecca-rabinowitz/the-uns-battle-with-ncds.

7. United Nations, Document A/66/L.1, "Political Declaration of the High-level Meeting of the General Assembly on the Prevention and Control of Non-communicable Diseases," September 16, 2011, pp. 3, 6, available at www.un.org/ga/search/view_doc.asp?symbol=A/66/L.1.

8. WHO, Executive Board Resolution 130.R7, "Prevention and Control of Non-communicable Diseases: Follow-up to the High-level Meeting of the United Nations

General Assembly on the Prevention and Control of Non-communicable Diseases," January 20, 2012, pp. 3–4, available at http://apps.who.int/gb/ebwha/pdf_files/EB130/B130_R7-en.pdf.

9. Thomas J. Bollyky, "The Path Forward on NCDs," CFR Expert Brief, September 22, 2011, available at www.cfr.org/health-and-disease/path-forward-ncds/p26006?cid=rss-expertbriefs-the_path_forward_on_ncds-092211.

10. National Public Radio, "Food Industry Pitted against Public Health at U.N. Summit," Shots Health Blog, September 20, 2011, available at www.npr.org/blogs/health/2011/09/20/140644556/food-industry-pitted-against-public-health-at-u-n-summit.

11. Rachel A. Nugent and Dean T. Jamison, "What Can a UN Health Summit Do?" *Science Translational Medicine*, 3 (2011): 1–3.

12. See, for example, Laurie Garrett, "So, What Was Accomplished? The UN and NCDs," The Garrett Update, September 2011, available at www.lauriegarrett.com/index.php/en/blog/3042/.

13. Charles Kenny, *Getting Better: Why Global Development Is Succeeding* (New York: Basic Books, 2011), 122, 125–26.

14. Ibid.; World Bank, "Health," Data Indicators, p. 2012, available at http://data.worldbank.org/topic/health.

15. Michael Maurice Engelgau et al., *Capitalizing on the Demographic Transition: Tackling Noncommunicable Diseases in South Asia* (Washington, DC: World Bank, 2011), 3.

16. Shaohua Chen and Martin Ravallion, "The Developing World Is Poorer than We Thought, But No Less Successful in the Fight against Poverty," *Quarterly Journal of Economics*, 125 (2010): 1601.

17. Andy Sumner, *Global Poverty and the New Bottom Billion: What If Three-Quarters of the World's Poor Live in Middle-Income Countries?* Institute of Development Studies Working Paper 349 (2010), 18.

18. Chunling Lu et al., "Public Financing of Health in Developing Countries: A Cross-National Systematic Analysis," *Lancet*, 375 (2010): 1375, 1379–82.

19. Ibid.; World Bank, "World Development Indicators (2008)," available at http://data.worldbank.org/products/data-books/WDI-2008. Overall, U.S. health spending in 1998 was $4,000 per person; Sub-Saharan African nations' spending constituted only $8 per person, with some countries spending as little as $2 per person.

20. Irina A. Nikolic, Anderson E. Stanciole, and Mikhail Zaydman, *Chronic Emergency: Why NCDs Matter* (Washington, DC: International Bank for Reconstruction and Development/World Bank, 2011), 6; Engelgau et al., *Capitalizing on the Demographic Transition*, 21.

21. Lawrence O. Gostin, "The 'Tobacco Wars'—Global Litigation Strategies," *JAMA*, 298 (2007): 2537–38.

22. Prabhat Jha et al., "Tobacco Addiction," in *Disease Control Priorities in Developing Countries*, ed. Dean T. Jamison et al. (Washington, DC: World Bank, 2006), 869–85.

23. See, e.g., Duff Wilson, "Tobacco Funds Shrink as Obesity Fight Intensifies," *New York Times*, July 27, 2010, available at www.nytimes.com/2010/07/28/health/policy/

28obesity.html; Thomas J. Bollyky, *Beyond Ratification: The Future of U.S. Engagement on International Tobacco Control* (Washington, DC: Center for Strategic and International Studies, 2010), 12–13.

24. International Centre for Trade and Sustainable Development, "Tobacco Company Files Claim against Uruguay over Labeling Laws," March 10, 2010, http://ictsd.org/i/news/bridgesweekly/71988/.

25. Katharine M. Esson and Stephen R. Leeder, *The Millennium Development Goals and Tobacco Control* (Geneva: WHO, 2004), xi.

26. Omar Shafey et al., *The Tobacco Atlas, Third Edition* (Atlanta: American Cancer Society, 2009), 30; WHO, "WHO Calls for Protection of Women and Girls from Tobacco," press release, May 24, 2010, available at www.who.int/mediacentre/news/releases/2010/women_tobacco_20100528/en/index.html.

27. Steven Allender et al., "Quantifying Urbanization as a Risk Factor for Noncommunicable Disease," *Journal of Urban Health*, 88 (2001): 906.

28. Tim Campbell and Alana Campbell, "Emerging Disease Burdens and the Poor in Cities of the Developing World," *Journal of Urban Health*, 84 (2007): 155.

29. Julie E. Fischer and Rebecca Katz, "The International Flow of Risk: The Governance of Health in an Urbanizing World," *Global Health Governance* 4 (2011): 2; Campbell and Campbell, "Emerging Disease Burdens," 159.

30. Fischer and Katz, "International Flow of Risk," 4.

31. WHO, *Global Status Report on Non-Communicable Diseases 2010* (Geneva: WHO, 2011), vii.

32. Ibid., 12.

33. Nikolic, Stanciole, and Zaydman, *Chronic Emergency*, 3.

34. WHO, *Global Status Report*, viii, 37; WHO, "WHO Maps Noncommunicable Disease Trends in All Countries," press release, September 14, 2011, available at www.who.int/mediacentre/news/releases/2011/NCDs_profiles_20110914/en/index.html.

35. Ibid., 10.

36. Ibid., 1.

37. "The Good News about Cancer in Developing Countries," *Lancet*, 378 (2011): 1605.

38. World Bank, *Toward a Healthy and Harmonious Life in China* (Washington, DC: World Bank, 2011), 3.

39. WHO, *Global Status Report*, 9.

40. Ibid., 1.

41. Nikolic, Stanciole, and Zaydman, *Chronic Emergency*, 6, 9–10.

42. Valentín Fuster and Bridget B. Kelly, eds., *Promoting Cardiovascular Health in the Developing World: A Critical Challenge to Achieve Global Health* (Washington, DC: National Academies Press, 2010), 1136–43; Robert Beaglehole et al., "UN High Level Meeting on Non-Communicable Diseases: Addressing Four Questions," *Lancet*, 378 (2011): 450.

43. Nikolic, Stanciole, and Zaydman, *Chronic Emergency*, 3–9.

44. David Bloom et al., *The Global Economic Burden of Non-Communicable Diseases* (Geneva: World Economic Forum, 2011), 29.

45. Amanda Glassman, "Global Chronic Disease: It's Not All about the Money for Once," *The Atlantic*, September 13, 2011, available at www.theatlantic.com/health/archive/2011/09/global-chronic-disease-its-not-all-about-the-money-for-once/244968/; Disease Control Priorities Project/World Bank, "Noncommunicable Diseases: Noncommunicable Diseases Now Account for a Majority of Deaths in Low- and Middle-Income Countries," July 2006, available at www.dcp2.org/file/58/DCPP-NCD.pdf.

46. Soeren Mattke et al., *Improving Access to Medicines for Non-Communicable Diseases in the Developing World* (Santa Monica: RAND Corporation, 2011), 17.

47. Ruth Levine, *Millions Saved: Proven Successes in Global Health* (Washington, DC: Center for Global Development, 2004).

48. WHO, *Report on the Global Tobacco Epidemic, 2011: Warning about the Dangers of Tobacco* (Geneva: WHO, 2011), 8; Bollyky, *Beyond Ratification*, 1.

49. Valentín Fuster and Bridget B. Kelly, eds., *Promoting Cardiovascular Health in the Developing World: A Critical Challenge to Achieve Global Health* (Washington, DC: National Academies Press, 2010), 73.

50. There are currently 174 parties to the FCTC, but one is the European Community, which is not a state. WHO, "Parties to the WHO Framework Convention on Tobacco Control," available at www.who.int/fctc/signatories_parties/en/index.html.

51. The acronym stands for: **M**onitor tobacco use and policies; **P**rotect people from second-hand smoke, **O**ffer help to quit; **W**arn about the dangers of tobacco; **E**nforce bans on advertising, promotion, and tobacco company sponsorship; and **R**aise taxes on tobacco products. See WHO, *Report on the Global Tobacco Epidemic, 2008: The MPOWER Package* (Geneva: WHO, 2008), 23.

52. U.S. Centers for Disease Control and Prevention (CDC), "Global Tobacco Surveillance System (GTSS)," available at www.cdc.gov/tobacco/global/gtss/index.htm; WHO, *Global Tobacco Epidemic*.

53. Bollyky, *Beyond Ratification*, 2.

54. Thomas J. Bollyky, "Forging a New Trade Policy on Tobacco," CFR Policy Innovation Memorandum No. 7, August 2011, available at www.cfr.org/trade/forging-new-trade-policy-tobacco/p25658.

55. Global Task Force on Expanded Access to Cancer Care and Control in Developing Countries, "The Partners in Health and Dana-Farber Cancer Institute Partnership," available at http://gtfccc.harvard.edu/icb/icb.do?keyword=k69586&pageid=icb.page342840.

Humanitarian Response in the Era of Global Mobile Information Technology / Valerie Amos

1. A video of the creation of this volunteer map is viewable at http://vimeo.com/9182869.

2. See (SBTF team member) Patrick Meier, "The [unexpected] Impact of the Libya Crisis Map and the Standby Volunteer Task Force," available at http://blog.standbytaskforce.com/sbtf-libya-impact/.

3. One of several accounts of the intervention can be found on the SBTF website: http://blog.standbytaskforce.com/unhcr-somalia-latest-results/.

4. Internews, *Dadaab, Kenya: Humanitarian Communications and Information Needs Assessment among Refugees in the Camps* (Washington, DC: Internews), available at www .internews.org/sites/default/files/resources/Dadaab2011-09-14.pdf.

5. Statement by WFP.

6. Linus Bengtsson, Xin Lu, Richard Garfield, Anna Thorson, and Johan von Schreeb, *Internal Population Displacement in Haiti: Preliminary Analyses of Movement Patterns of Digicel Mobile Phones: 1 January to 11 March 2010* (Karolinska Institute and Columbia University), available at http://haiti.humanitarianresponse.info/LinkClick.aspx ?fileticket=ZPH8pFFkMnU%3D&tabid=149&mid=1045.

7. See for example Concern Worldwide, Oxford Policy Management, and the Partnership for Research in International Affairs and Development, *New Technologies in Cash Transfer Programming and Humanitarian Assistance* (Oxford: Cash Learning Partnership, 2011), 57.

Disasters and the Media / Jeremy Toye

1. For North America see the Audit Bureau of Circulations (ABC) website (www .accessabc.com) and the related ABC sites for other countries.

2. Pliny's account of the disaster makes clear warning signs that Vesuvius was about to erupt were ignored, and no help came. See Andrew Wallace-Hadrill, "Pompeii: Portents of Disaster," BBC.co.uk, last modified March 29, 2011, available at www .bbc.co.uk/history/ancient/romans/pompeii_portents_01.shtml.

3. News of the assassination in 1865 took its time to reach the rest of the world—a steamship voyage across the Atlantic. The laying of the first transatlantic cable and subsequent global network made information flow almost instantaneous.

4. See www.parliament.uk.

5. See "Issue Brief: Ethiopian Famine 25th Anniversary," One.org, available at http://one.org/c/us/issuebrief/3127/.

6. See the Museum of Broadcast Communications (www.museum.tv), an archive of TV footage which features news of Vietnam War.

7. The video won the George Polk award for videography in 2009. See Robert McFadden, "Times Reporter Held by Taliban Is among Polk Award Winners," *New York Times*, February 16, 2010.

8. Between August 6 and 10, 2011, several districts of London and provincial cities were hit by riots involving looting and arson, with the police seemingly unable or unwilling to intervene.

9. Copies of the video can be found on the web, but their distribution was condemned at the time.

10. Reporters without Borders (www.rsf.org) said sixty-seven journalists were killed in 2011 alone. See "2011: 67 Journalists Killed," Reporters without Borders,

available at http://en.rsf.org/press-freedom-barometer-journalists-killed.html
?annee=2011.

11. See http://www.rt.com and others.

12. "Television? The word is half Greek and half Latin. No good can come of it."
Attributed to Scott by various sources, in slightly different forms.

13. Scottish Television's Roy Thomson, quoted by www.news.bbc.co.uk, available
at http://news.bbc.co.uk/2/hi/entertainment/1229805.stm.

14. In a Mozambique community where I have worked on a tiny community support scheme, we sent a messenger on foot for several hours to deliver a phone SIM card
to a village chief so he could discuss the next stage in building classrooms. See www
.mandawilderness.org.

15. See www.guardian.co.uk/katine.

16. Conversation with the author, 2011.

17. Newspaper Death Watch (newspaperdeathwatch.com) listed fourteen U.S.
metropolitan dailies that had closed by early 2012, including the Rocky Mountain News
and the Albuquerque Tribune.

18. See report on online versus traditional advertising on readwriteweb.com.

19. See the Huffington Post (www.huffingtonpost.com) and others. The fact that
over 70 million people watched a thirty-minute video produced by the hitherto little-
known charity Invisible Children provoked controversy, though it was unclear whether
it would help or hinder the search for the leader of a ruthless band of killers operating
in Central Africa.

20. There are surprisingly few truly international agencies: Associated Press, Reuters, Agence France Presse, and Kyodo are the main ones.

21. When I asked the Information Minister of Ethiopia why he never seemed to
have any information to impart, he replied with a smirk that it was his job to collect
information, not to hand it out to the likes of me.

22. I asked a government spokesman for an update on a bird flu outbreak: "Eighty
percent of the poultry tested was unaffected," he said loftily. "So 20 percent had bird
flu?" I said. "That is not an acceptable question," he railed. To be fair, it was a training
session, and once he had calmed down, he accepted that it might have been better
handled.

23. Bolton speaking on February 3, 1994. See "John Bolton in His Own Words:
Bush's UN Ambassador Nominee Condemns United Nations," Democracy Now, last
modified March 31, 2005, available at www.democracynow.org/2005/3/31/john_bolton_
in_his_own_words.

24. It was originally the United Nations International Children's Emergency
Fund.

25. See www.wfp.org/about/executive-director.

26. See www.unicef.org.

27. See www.wfp.com/molly.

28. The fashion chain Benetton courted further controversy when it showed images of such mutilations in a series of advertisements.

29. Journalists at a MediaTrain conference in Khartoum readily agreed that naming and showing the faces of child soldiers involved in a Justice and Equality Movement rebel attack could lead to reprisals against them and their families by both sides in the conflict.

30. One supposedly genuine NGO in East Africa repeatedly sends invitations to conferences that don't exist, working a scam that echoes the infamous e-mails from alleged Nigerians offering million-dollar payouts in return for bank account details.

31. See conservapedia.com/climategate.

32. The huge unused stocks of Tamiflu in some countries that were built up in response to the bird and swine flu scares are testimony to how that reaction can itself be excessive.

33. See Steven Ross, *Toward New Understandings: Journalists and Humanitarian Relief Coverages* (San Francisco: Fritz Institute, 2004), available at www.fritzinstitute.org/PDFs/Case-Studies/Media_study_excSum.pdf.

34. See the Governance and Social Development Resource Center (www.gsdrc.org).

35. See "Burma's Aung San Suu Kyi Makes Landmark Campaign Speech," BBC.co.uk, last modified March 14, 2012, available at http:// bbc.co.uk/news/world-asia-17363329.

36. See "Schindler's Factory in Krakow," Krakow-Info, available at www.krakow-info.com/schindler.htm.

Toward a Culture of Safety and Resilience / Irina Bokova

1. See United Nations International Strategy for Disaster Reduction (UNISDR), *Global Assessment Report on Disaster Risk Reduction: Risk, and Poverty in a Changing Climate* (Geneva: UNISDR, 2009).

2. Summary statement from the Japan-UNESCO/UNU Symposium on "The Great East Japan Tsunami on 11 March 2011 and Tsunami Warning Systems: Policy Perspectives," February 16–17, 2012, United Nations University, Tokyo, Japan.

3. Statement by Michaëlle Jean made at Columbia University at the launch of the UNESCO's *Education for All Global Monitoring Report: The Hidden Crisis, Armed Conflict and Education* (Paris: UNESCO, 2011).

4. Central Emergency Respond Fund (CERF), *CERF Two Year Evaluation—Final Report* (New York: CERF, 2008).

5. UNESCO, *Education for All Global Monitoring Report: The Hidden Crisis, Armed Conflict and Education* (Paris: UNESCO, 2011).

6. In China, an earthquake in May 2008 affected Mount Qingcheng and the Dujiangyan Irrigation System and the Sichuan Giant Panda Sanctuaries. In Haiti, an earthquake in January 2010 caused structural damage to the National History Park—Citadel, Sans Souci, Ramiers. The Historic Center of Jacmel was also heavily impacted. In Iran, an earthquake in December 2003 destroyed the Citadel of Bam (Arg-e-Bam). In Thailand, floods in July 2011 inundated the Historic City of Ayutthaya.

7. See, for Instance, UNESCO, *Managing Disaster Risks for World Heritage* (Paris: UNESCO, 2010). Available at http://whc.unesco.org/uploads/activities/documents/activity-630-1.pdf.

8. UNESCO, "Donation for Safeguarding the Borobudur Temple Compounds" (Paris: UNESCO, 2012).

9. See Johan Rockström et al., "A Safe Operating Space for Humanity," *Nature* 461 (2009): 472–75.

10. UN Secretary General's High-level Panel on Global Sustainability, *Resilient People, Resilient Planet: A Future Worth Choosing* (New York: UN, 2012).

11. World Commission on Culture and Development, *Our Creative Diversity* (Paris: UNESCO, 1996).

Education and Disaster Management / Kevin M. Cahill, M.D., and Alexander van Tulleken, M.D.

1. James Fearon, "The Rise of Emergency Relief Aid," in *Humanitarianism in Question: Politics, Power, Ethics*, ed. Michael N. Barnett and Thomas George Weiss (Ithaca: Cornell University Press, 2008), 303.

2. Alexander De Waal, *Famine Crimes: Politics and the Disaster Relief Industry in Africa* (London: African Rights & the International African Institute, 1997).

3. Peter Salama and Les Roberts, "Evidence-Based Interventions in Complex Emergencies," *Lancet* 365.9474 (2005): 1848.

4. See Issue 48 (October 2010) of *Humanitarian Exchange Magazine* (published by the Humanitarian Practice Network), which focuses on the response to the January 2010 earthquake in Haiti.

5. For more information on Fordham University's Institute of International Humanitarian Affairs, visit www.fordham.edu/iiha.

6. Kevin M. Cahill, *The University and Humanitarian Assistance*, Occasional Paper No. 4, January 18, 2008, Institute of International Humanitarian Affairs, Fordham University.

7. Kevin M. Cahill, *A Bridge to Peace* (New York: Haymarket Doyma Inc., 1988).

8. Kevin M. Cahill, "Training for Humanitarian Assistance," in *Basics of International Humanitarian Missions*, ed. Kevin M. Cahill (New York: Fordham University Press, 2003), 49–58.

9. For more information about the Jesuit Universities Humanitarian Action Network, visit www.juhanproject.org.

Capitalizing on Travel and Tourism in Preparing for Trouble / Richard Gordon

1. The United Nations International Strategy for Disaster Reduction (UNISDR) definition of a disaster is a "serious disruption of the functioning of a community or a society

involving widespread human, material, economic or environmental losses and impacts, which exceeds the ability of the affected community or society to cope using its own resources" (2009 *UNISDR Terminology on Disaster Risk Reduction* [Geneva: UNISDR, 2009], 9).

2. See www.unisdr.org.

3. UNISDR, *Hyogo Framework for Action 2005–2015: Building the Resilience of Nations and Communities to Disasters: Mid-Term Review 2010–2011* (Geneva: UNISDR, 2011), available at www.unisdr.org/we/inform/publications/18197.

4. UNISDR, *Words into Action: A Guide for Implementing the Hyogo Framework* (Geneva: UNISDR, 2007), available at www.unisdr.org/files/594_10382.pdf.

5. Ibid., 10.

6. UNWTO, *Technical Manual: Concepts, Definitions and Classifications for Tourism Statistics* (Madrid: UNTWO, 1995), available at http://pub.unwto.org/WebRoot/Store/Shops/Infoshop/Products/1033/1033-1.pdf.

7. Macintosh and Goeldner, *Definition of Tourism*, available at http://travelandtourisms.com/search/macintosh-and-goeldner-definition-of-tourism-1986/.

8. John G. C. Kester, "2011 International Tourism Results and Prospects for 2012," presentation given at UNWTO News Conference, Madrid, January 16, 2012, available at http://dtxtq4w60xqpw.cloudfront.net/sites/all/files/pdf/unwto_hq_fitur12_jk_2pp_0.pdf.

9. Ibid.

10. Ibid.

11. Ibid.

12. Impact Forecasting's *Annual Global Climate and Catastrophe Report* (Chicago: Impact Forecasting, 2012) reveals that 2011 was one of the most active years on record for natural catastrophes, with 253 separate events, generating a record total economic loss of $435 billion. The total insured loss from natural catastrophes during 2011 ($107 billion) was the second highest on record, surpassed only by the $120 billion insured loss witnessed in 2005, of which $90 billion resulted from the major hurricanes Katrina, Rita, and Wilma. This also marks a more than 280 percent increase from insured losses seen in 2010. These insured financial losses and other uninsured costs also resulted in many tourism-related businesses being liquidated or losing profits and brand image through not having adequate disaster and emergency policies in place.

13. Interview with Jean Marc Flambert, who was with the Sri Lanka Tourist Board during the 2004 tsunami.

14. Interpol Standing Committee on DVI, Resolution No. AGN/65/Res/13.

15. For Agenda 21 see www.un.org/esa/dsd/agenda21/.

16. See United Nations Environment Programme and the UNTWO, *Making Tourism More Sustainable: A Guide for Policy Makers* (Paris: 2005), available at www.unep.fr/shared/publications/pdf/DTIx0592xPA-TourismPolicyEN.pdf.

17. Presentation by Masato Takamatsu, CEO, Japan Tourism Marketing Company, to Australian Emergency Management Institute, September 2011.

Business in an Age of Emergency / Richard Branson

1. Center for Research on the Epidemiology of Disease (CRED), *Annual Disaster Statistical Review 2010—The Numbers and Trends* (Brussels: CRED, 2011), available at www.cred.be/sites/default/files/ADSR_2010.pdf. See also CRED and United Nations International Strategy for Disaster Reduction, "Earthquakes Caused the Deadliest Disasters in the Past Decade" (press release), available at http://reliefweb.int/node/343202.

2. See www.unhcr.org/4ef1ec326.html.

3. About half represents assistance disbursed as of March 2012 (53 percent). Donors have also provided Haiti with about $1 billion in debt relief. See UN Office of the Special Envoy for Haiti, *International Assistance Tracker* (New York: UN Office of the Special Envoy, 2012), available at www.haitispecialenvoy.org/assistance-tracker/.

4. Oxfam, *Haiti: The Slow Road the Reconstruction; Two Years after the Earthquake* (Oxford: Oxfam, 2012), available at www.oxfam.org/en/policy/haiti-slow-road-reconstruction.

5. William Paton, *Philanthropic Grantmaking for Disasters: Lessons Learned at the Conrad Hilton Foundation* (Los Angeles: Conrad N. Hilton Foundation, 2011) and "Disaster Giving," Center on Philanthropy at Indiana University, available at www.philanthropy.iupui.edu/research/disaster.aspx.

6. Oxfam, *Haiti*.

7. United Nations International Strategy for Disaster Reduction, available at www.unisdr.org/we/advocate/sustainable-development.

8. United Nations International Strategy for Disaster Reduction Secretariat (UNISDR) (www.unisdr.org).

9. Global Humanitarian Forum, *Human Impact Report: Climate Change—The Anatomy of a Silent Crisis* (Geneva: Global Humanitarian Forum, 2009), available at www.bb.undp.org/uploads/file/pdfs/energy_environment/CC%20human%20impact%20report.pdf.

10. Paton, *Philanthropic Grantmaking*.

Terror, Transformed: A Financier's Journey into Social Entrepreneurship / Michael Pollack

1. Plato, *The Republic*, bk. VII, sect. 518c.

2. Indian Government Survey, 2008–9.

3. Copal Partners Research, *India's Charity Sector: An Overview and Analytical Approach* (Delhi: Copal Partners Research, 2006).

4. Educate Girls, *Impact Study CLT* (Mumbai: Reliable Business Centre, 2010).

5. Anton Chekov, "Gooseberries," 1898.

H.E. NASSIR ABDULAZIZ AL-NASSER is the President of the United Nations General Assembly (Sixty-Sixth Session). Prior to his appointment as President, he had served the United Nations as Permanent Representative of Qatar, President of the Security Council, and in other leadership capacities since 1998.

VALERIE AMOS is the Under-Secretary-General and Emergency Relief Coordinator for the United Nations Office for the Coordination of Humanitarian Affairs (OCHA). She has previously served as a Minister in the British Government, and has been active for over thirty years on the promotion of human rights, social justice, and equality on the African continent.

IRINA BOKOVA is the Director-General of the United Nation Education, Scientific and Cultural Organization (UNESCO). She formerly served as Ambassador of the Republic of Bulgaria to France and Monaco, Personal Representative of the Bulgarian President to the Organisation Internationale de la Francophonie, and Permanent Delegate to UNESCO from 2005 to 2009.

THOMAS J. BOLLYKY is the Senior Fellow for global health, economics, and development at the Council on Foreign Relations. He is also an adjunct professor of law at Georgetown University, a consultant to the

Bill and Melinda Gates Foundation, and a health policy advisor to the Clinton Global Initiative.

RICHARD BRANSON is the founder of Virgin Records, which has expanded into the Virgin Group of more than 400 companies. He is a financial "Founder" of the South African humanitarian group, The Elders, and has established the Branson School of Entrepreneurship in Johannesburg.

FLAVIA BUSTREO, M.D., is the Deputy Director of the Partnership for Maternal, Newborn and Child Health (PMNCH) at the World Health Organization (WHO). She has served as a Senior Public Health Specialist responsible for the WHO-World Bank partnership for child health management and participates in the UN Taskforce on Millennium Development Goals 4 and 5 to reduce maternal and child mortality.

KEVIN M. CAHILL, M.D., is University Professor and Director of the Institute of International Humanitarian Affairs at Fordham University. He has served as the Chief Advisor on Humanitarian and Public Health Issues to three Presidents of the United Nations General Assembly. He is the Director of the Tropical Disease Center of Lenox Hill hospital in New York City.

THOMAS FRESTON is a principal in Firefly3 LLC and the Chairman of the Board of the ONE Foundation. He is the former CEO of MTV Networks and former President and CEO of Viacom Inc.

RICHARD GORDON is the Director of the Bournemouth University Disaster Management Centre. He has designed, coordinated, and delivered disaster management projects in the Middle East, West Africa, South and East Asia, Eastern Europe, and the United States.

MASOOD HYDER has worked for the UN World Food Programme (WFP) as Representative to Sudan, as Resident Coordinator for North

Korea and as WFP Representative to the Bretton Woods Institutions. He now teaches a graduate course on humanitarian action at the Maxwell School, Syracuse University.

RONAN MURPHY served two terms as Director General of Irish Aid. He also served as Senior Advisor to Mary Robinson when she was UN High Commissioner for Human Rights. He is currently Chief Operating Officer of the Mary Robinson Foundation—Climate Justice. His book, *Inside Irish Aid*, will be published in 2012 by Liffey Press, Dublin.

MICHAEL POLLACK is the Founder and President of the SCA Charitable Foundation. He is also a managing partner of the Pollack Holdings Investment Firm.

DOMINICK SALVATORE is Distinguished Professor of Economics at Fordham University. He is the former President of the North American Economic and Finance Association (NAEFA) and the International Trade and Finance Association (ITFA), and serves as a Consultant to the United Nations, the World Bank, the International Monetary Fund, and the Economic Policy Institute.

JEREMY TOYE is a founding member of MediaTrain. He has designed and delivered over eighty workshops around the world, concentrating particularly on UN staff at all levels. He was a Reuters correspondent and international manager for twenty-eight years, working in some sixty countries. He served as an FAO press officer in Indonesia in the aftermath of the Asian Tsunami.

ALEXANDER VAN TULLEKEN, M.D., is the Helen Hamlyn Senior Fellow at Fordham University's Institute of International Humanitarian Affairs (IIHA). He has worked for MDM, Merlin, and the World Health Organization in humanitarian crises around the world.

MARGARETA WAHLSTROM is the Special Representative of the Secretary-General for Disaster Risk Reduction for the United Nations and Head of the United Nations International Strategy for Disaster Reduction (UNISDR). She has served as Deputy Emergency Relief Co-ordinator and Assistant Secretary-General for Humanitarian Affairs, OCHA.

The Center for International
Humanitarian Cooperation and
the Institute of International
Humanitarian Affairs

The Center for International Humanitarian Cooperation (CIHC) is a public charity founded by a small group of international diplomats and physicians who believe that health and other humanitarian endeavors sometimes provide the only common ground for initiating dialogue, understanding, and cooperation among people and nations shattered by war, civil conflicts, and ethnic violence. The CIHC has sponsored symposia and published books, including *Silent Witnesses, A Directory of Somali Professionals*, and *Clearing the Fields: Solutions to the Global Land Mine Crisis*, as well as the International Humanitarian Book Series of Fordham University Press listed at the end of this book.

The Center and its Directors have been deeply involved in trying to alleviate the wounds of war in many areas. A CIHC amputee center in northern Somalia was developed as a model for a simple, rapid, and inexpensive program that could be replicated in other war zones. In the former Yugoslavia, the CIHC was active in prisoner and hostage release and in legal assistance for human and political rights violations, and facilitated discussions between combatants.

The CIHC collaborated with Fordham University in 2001 to foster close links between academia and humanitarian field operations, creating an Institute of International Humanitarian Affairs (IIHA). Its flagship course is the International Diploma in Humanitarian Assistance (IDHA), which is offered three times a year in different locations throughout the world. The IDHA has graduated more than 1,800 leaders in the humanitarian world from 133 nations, representing all agencies of the United Nations and major nongovernmental organizations (NGOs) around the world. The IIHA at Fordham University in New York offers a graduate Masters Degree in International Humanitarian Action (MIHA) and an undergraduate International Humanitarian Affairs Minor program. The IIHA also offers specialized training courses for humanitarian negotiators, international human rights lawyers, and mental health workers in war zones. Please visit www.fordham.edu/iiha.

The Center has provided staff support in recent years in crisis management in Iraq, East Timor, Aceh, Kosovo, Palestine, Albania, Lebanon, Pakistan, Somalia, Kenya, and other trouble spots. The Center has been afforded full Economic and Social Council (ECOSOC) consultative status at the United Nations. In the United States, it is a fully approved public charity. The Directors of the CIHC serve as the Advisory Board of the IIHA. The President of the CIHC is the University Professor and Director of the Institute, the CIHC Humanitarian Programs Director is Visiting Professor at the IIHA, and another CIHC Director is the Diplomat in Residence at Fordham University.

Directors
Kevin M. Cahill, M.D., President
Boutros Boutros-Ghali
Francis Deng
Richard Goldstone
Helen Hamlyn
Peter Hansen
Eoin O'Brien, M.D.
Joseph A. O'Hare, S.J.
David Owen
Peter Tarnoff

INDEX